YOUR PAIN
IS NOT
A WASTE

Finding Answers, Hope, and
the Meaning of Life in the Midst of Pain

YOUR PAIN
IS NOT
A WASTE

Finding Answers, Hope, and
the Meaning of Life in the Midst of Pain

D. N. Grace

Books By Grace LLC
Winter Springs, Florida

Disclaimer. *YOUR PAIN IS NOT A WASTE* tells the story of its author. Treatments mentioned in this book belong to the author's case and her unique experience. The author's failed treatment, the side effects, and reactions do not necessarily mean this will happen to you too. This book is not meant to provide medical information or advice or to recommend specific treatment protocol. For information about your treatment, always refer to your own treatment team.

YOUR PAIN IS NOT A WASTE: Finding Answers, Hope, and the Meaning of Life in the Midst of Pain

Library of Congress Control Number: 2020911547
ISBN: 978-1-7352520-0-1 paperback
ISBN: 978-1-7352520-1-8 hardback
ISBN: 978-1-7352520-2-5 ebook
ISBN: 978-1-7352520-3-2 audiobook

Cover designed by Shadi Maher
Author picture courtesy of Remon Manssour
Translation of Neveen's and May's chapters by Sandy Saleeb
Writing consultant/editor Judy Sheer Watters, Hearts Need Art
Editor Maxwell Mitzel
Made possible by the Dear Jack Foundation

Contact the author at DNGrace@dngrace.com
Website: www.DNGrace.com
Facebook: https://www.facebook.com/YourPainIsNotAWaste/
Instagram: @D.N.Grace

This book was printed in the United States of America.

Table of Contents

Dedication

To all who are facing pain,
fighting a battle of survival.
You are Not Alone.

To my husband and best friend—
In sickness and in health . . . Every time I
said to myself, *love can't give anymore,* you
proved that I was sooo wrong. You always
had and still have more love that you freely
pour into me. Your love is a renewable
river—deep, fresh, and enduring.

Introduction

Since I thought about writing this book, I was praying day and night for the person who will read it. I know everything happens for a reason. I believe this book will find you. You are the right person for this book.

I am a very simple girl. My life was not simple or easy even before I had cancer. But my heart always searched for God. I never blamed Him in anything, but all the time I wanted to know the reason for what was happening to me.

I care a lot about my achievements, goals, and having a timeframe for everything even in my relation with God. I used to consider my illness and pain as lost time. However, I have learned that God only cares about *you*, and He can do wonders with *you*, but in His own timing.

This book is not just about sickness and pain. It's about how He keeps working in your life to peel off all the fake things that create a shell around you. He does this in order to form and show the best you that you can possibly be.

Remember: It's not about what you want to achieve. It's about what God wants from you and for you. Are you willing to let Him work within you?

Pain is a Part of Life

Today I decided not to waste my pain.
I will learn the lesson—I know, oh God, that you
let this happen to me.
Is this just because you trust me? You count on me,
and I accept it.
I know that someday, I will find the reason.
Until that day comes, I promise you, God,
I will never waste my pain.

My diary entry on November 1, 2017

CHAPTER 1
Dream School or Worst Nightmare?
Dalia

February 2017

I'm still young; nothing bad will happen to me.

These were my thoughts during a time when I began to feel that something was wrong inside me. There was so much pain in my left side; my lower back was killing me, but I had no time for that, and my part-time job did not provide any insurance. At first, I believed it was just exhaustion, that working too much and studying too hard was the source of the pain.

But it was getting worse. My face became so pale; I fainted many times at work. But I didn't tell my husband, because I didn't want him to get worried or frustrated. I needed him to focus on his studies, his work, and I didn't think it was a big deal. I just needed some rest.

My name is Dalia, and this is my story. I see myself as a normal woman in her 20s, active, ambitious, and hardworking. I love my family, my husband, and my friends, and my passion is serving others.

Throughout 2016, before my diagnosis, I had been working two jobs, as my husband, Remon, had been studying for his pharmacy license and working part-time. We support each other, so we were happy with this arrangement.

I also was studying as well as working. I've had a dream since before I moved to the United States. I served Sunday school kids and high school age adolescents in Egypt. I cared about them a lot, and when I listened to their problems, I really wanted to give them professional spiritual and biblical advice.

When I moved to America, I finally found my dream school: Reformed Theological Seminary in Orlando (RTS). It could give me the academic Christian counseling study that I had been searching for my whole life. I was so excited. I decided I would do whatever it took to get accepted into this school and get my master's degree in theological counseling.

It had everything I'd ever wanted.

I had read a lot about this school. I worked in the morning, studied at night, and wrote my essays in whatever spare time I had left because I really wanted them to choose *me*. I knew there were hundreds of students applying for this school every single year, but the college only chose a select few. I had to convince them through my writing. I focused all my energy on winning them over.

I had to.

The school had many conditions for foreigners, but I *needed* this. I could do it. This was my dream, my calling, my purpose—I knew God would be happy with me for this study and service.

My dream was—and is still—to have my master's degree in counseling. I would work as hard as I possibly could to reach this, no matter what.

The college sent me an email stating that they were interested in my file; they wanted me to be at orientation and have some interviews with the professors in the school. That same day, my manager at work told me they wanted me to do another interview. They wanted to promote me to a different department, which meant I would get a raise in my salary. That was a day to remember! I was so happy. I felt like everything was exactly as I had planned. Life was opening its arms and showering me with blessings.

While I celebrated by jumping and laughing from the bottom of my heart, I fainted. Everything got dark; the pain was unbearable.

I called my sister. She insisted I tell my husband that I had to go to the hospital immediately.

I called Remon and told him what happened, then I drove home and waited for him to return from work.

All I could think about was my orientation; I had to be fully prepared. *What should I wear? What questions will they ask? I have to study; I have to prepare.* I didn't even think for a second about my health situation because I was so sure my pain would pass.

While we waited at the hospital's reception, I told Remon how excited I was about the promotion, the orientation, and the interview for the next day.

They called my name. We met the nurse, and he asked me how I felt. I told him I felt dizzy, fatigued, and even fainted at work. He said that he would give me a painkiller and send me home.

But at that moment, my husband interfered. He didn't agree with what the nurse said; I remember he was so mad, so furious. He told the nurse he wouldn't leave this hospital until they knew what was going on with me, that he needed to meet the doctor, that I should have scans done.

The nurse relented.

When we met the doctor, she ordered some

scans for me. They'd find what was causing the pain.

But the pain, the hospital, none of that was on my mind. I kept telling Remon I really wanted to go home early because I had my orientation tomorrow morning. They kept transferring me through different scans, different rooms, over and over again. The six hours felt like eternity, and I needed it to go faster.

I looked into my husband's eyes, and I could feel how worried he was. I started to get anxious. Finally, the doctor returned, shouting at the nurses saying, "Nobody touch her side or move her." Then she sat beside my bed, a sad look in her eyes, and quietly told me that I had a very serious issue in my abdomen: my spleen was abnormally large and could explode at any moment. It had lots of blood cysts on it, which made my situation even more dangerous. But this hospital was not prepared for big surgeries, so they would have to transfer me to the main hospital. I needed immediate surgery.

"I will call one of the best surgeons I know," she said. "One who can perform this type of dangerous and sensitive surgery."

But I wasn't processing any of this. I was sure she was mistaken. And at some point, I couldn't hear anything she was saying despite seeing her lips moving.

When she finished, she asked me if I was okay with what she was suggesting.

I said to her, "With what?"

She answered that they were going to transfer me to the main hospital because I needed immediate surgery.

I remember that my response to her was that I had my orientation tomorrow, that I needed my discharge papers because it was dawn now. I needed to change and prepare for the orientation.

She was shocked by my answer, rather taken aback by my priorities, and restated how dire the situation was. She asked me if this school was even more valuable than my own life.

I started to question why I was so obsessed, with this school, this degree, that I would risk my own health, my own well-being to do so, even if it would quite literally kill me.

CHAPTER 2
The Beginning of Distress
Remon

December 2016

I was traveling to work when my manager called me to say that she had exceeded the limit of allocated schedule hours and had to cancel my shifts till the new year which was the following week and until then I could not work. I parked, and for a moment, it felt like everything in my life was collapsing. I was impatiently waiting for that day's shift to end because I only had seven hours left to work this year to be eligible for health insurance next year. I had worked the whole year, the maximum number of hours I could get, picked up every extra shift along with studying for my pharmacist license.

I hoped so much that we would be able to get health insurance this year. I knew my wife was not feeling well, but we couldn't go to the doctor because we didn't have insurance.

I told my manager I needed this shift and I was hoping to get benefits next year and asked if there was anything she could do. She told me she could make some phone calls and call me back, but in the meantime, I couldn't work.

As I waited, all sorts of thoughts stirred in my mind. I didn't know exactly what I was going to do if I didn't get health insurance. I needed to take my wife to a doctor. I worked and studied while my wife worked as much as she could. She also studied at the same time, but neither of us had insurance.

A few minutes later, my manager called and said that I could work. She was brief and didn't explain much, but she had figured something out.

I drove back to work that day. It was a seven-hour shift that completed my hours to get health benefits. I smiled all day out of relief, accomplishment, and gratefulness.

February 2017

A couple of weeks later, I received our insurance cards in the mail.

I knew my wife was tired all the time, but she was trying to power through. Both of us believed it was due to her overworking. Dalia had applied for a master's degree in counseling at RTS, and her application was accepted. She felt over the clouds as her dream came ever closer to being a reality.

I thought it might be a good idea to get her a chiropractor gift card for Valentine's Day. She felt tired all the time. I thought a good chiropractor session might make her feel better, but the reality was far different than what I had hoped for.

When Dalia went to see the chiropractor, the doctor couldn't even touch her. She had terrible pain in her abdomen and pelvis. The doctor couldn't perform any manipulations while she had this pain. They told her this was beyond their field of expertise. The chiropractor ordered an MRI scan to determine what was wrong.

When Dalia came back home, I was a bit surprised. I didn't expect things to be this bad.

Now, we would need to have an MRI done. It seemed as though everything took so much time. I felt it had taken me forever to book a chiropractor, then forever to find an MRI appointment, and forever to get the results back, even though we did all that in one week. Patience is not my best attribute. I tend to worry so much and usually try to react even if there's nothing I can do. The MRI results showed that she had something wrong with her spleen.

The chiropractor didn't wait for us to visit the office. She called Dalia while l was at work and told her she needed to take her MRI results and go see a specialist because it was extremely serious.

Sunday
The day before her RTS interview day, Dalia

called me from home and told me that she had passed out at work. She needed to go to the hospital.

She had resisted any sort of hospital visits before this due to her fears about preparing for her orientation and her interview, yet we couldn't wait anymore. I took her to the emergency room and was surprised that she didn't resist. Perhaps it was the pain.

I remember that night. Dalia didn't want to spend the night at the emergency room because she had interviews at the seminary the next morning. But with passing out at work and the terrible pain, she had no choice.

We knew there was something wrong with her spleen. We waited, filled out the forms, and then took her to the triage nurse.

The triage nurse usually asks about medical history and screens patients for domestic violence or abuse, and they prefer the patient to be alone to speak freely. Because I am a pharmacist, I knew that, but I didn't remember any of this at that time.

I went to the room with Dalia, answering all the questions before she did. The nurse gave me this look, likely thinking I had done something wrong and was trying to cover it up. That was long before our multiple visits there, before they started to know us very well. But at this time, I wasn't thinking at all. It was so terrifying and stressful—how could I think clearly?

As they performed test after test and scan after scan, all I can remember is that we were both so cold. We were shaking, but I don't know if it was the room temperature or the anxiety and worry about what they might tell us.

With every passing minute, I started to worry more and more. When the doctor finally returned, she told us that Dalia's blood work was bad; her hemoglobin was seven, maybe less, where a normal range should be 13.5-15. And her spleen was so enlarged that she required immediate surgery. They would admit her to the hospital until they could get the surgery scheduled.

Dalia refused profusely; She had her interviews the next day, and under no circumstances would she miss them. I was freaking out because of everything that was happening. They finally let us go home, as the small hospital wasn't equipped to deal with such a surgery, but they booked us an appointment at the main hospital for Wednesday.

Three days.

That's how long we would need to wait.

A lot could go wrong in three days.

"Trust in the Lord with all your heart, and do not lean on your own understanding.
In all your ways acknowledge him, and he will make straight your paths."
Proverbs 3:5-6

CHAPTER 3

Can You Control Everything?
Dalia

March 2017

Life often puts us in difficult situations. Some of them are beyond our control. We are then surprised that life is not all rosy, that we truly are not in control.

In my case, I decided to go on with my plans, denying the fact that I was sick. *Maybe what happened will postpone my plans or even cancel them; I am not prepared for this.*

I left the hospital to get ready for the orientation. My husband drove me to the RTS seminary; he was so worried about my health. After the orientation, I had four interviews. I was doing good until I felt dizzy and too exhausted. I fainted, so they called my husband, and he took me back to the hospital. Remon was so worried. I started to feel anxious, and the pain was indescribable.

At the hospital, they checked everything again for the second time in two days. Finally, they said I could go home, but this time, be very careful, rest, and keep the main hospital appointment.

Two days later, around 3:00 or 4:00 a.m., I woke screaming with pain. Remon knew my spleen could rupture anytime and could cost me my life. He decided to take me straight to the main hospital in Orlando as we had already booked a surgery appointment with them. As we drove to the hospital, I tried to calm him, but I couldn't because I was scared and in so much pain. I started to think about all the possibilities if my spleen ruptured. *Will I die right away? What about my husband, my family, and friends?* For the first time in my life, I felt death was close. My heart beat so fast.

When we arrived at the hospital, I remember that they were scared and confused when they saw me. One nurse was so nervous trying to put in an IV. Several times she tried but no success. I was so quiet through it all. I tried to calm the nurse and Remon.

They retrieved the scans results. One of the doctors said, "I see blood cysts over your spleen, and one of them may have already ruptured causing this pain. I don't know if we have time to save you until the surgery."

When he said that, I was so concerned about Remon. I looked at him; he couldn't take it, and he fell on the floor beside my bed. At this moment, I felt that we were both miserable, helpless, and lonely. After less than a minute, another doctor came to tell us that nothing had ruptured yet, but we had to be very careful until they performed the surgery.

I stayed in the hospital for five days before my operation since my body was so weak. I had to get iron and blood transfusions. Remon was so worried and anxious because every delay in my surgery could cost me my life.

All my family lived in Egypt. They were so depressed, as they could not be with me. They kept calling Remon asking him too many questions, and that added more pressure onto him. They got angry with him if he didn't answer. And he couldn't tell them all the details because he didn't want them to get more depressed or worried.

I had my spleen removed on March 14, 2017. The pain was so bad that I was hospitalized for ten days after the surgery. My surgeon and the nurses kept saying that for me to be alive was a miracle. They kept describing how difficult my surgery was and how my condition was very bad.

Remon stayed with me day and night; he wasn't thinking about his work or even his license. I asked him many times to go home even for one day. I told him, "You have to concentrate on your studies; that's your future."

I remember his answer to me.

"I have no future if you are not with me; you are my future. Staying with you is more valuable than any license I could ever get, any success I could ever achieve."

When he said that, I felt how lucky I was—how amazing his love was for me. I wanted to live—to spend more time with my husband. I was so thankful the surgeon could save my life and the only thing I kept asking myself was *why am I still alive. Is my life that important and valuable?*

When I got home, I found my friends from church had prepared meals for me. They decided to help me until I got better. One of them, Mays, came to be my best friend. She was a blessing in my life in every way you could imagine. After I came home, Mays was there for me every single day until I started to do my normal activities without help. We found that we have so much in common.

When I started to feel better, I looked at my life and my relationship with God, Remon, my family, and friends differently. I searched for a deeper meaning to my life. Even my prayers were different than before; I felt that life is short and anything could happen so I had to be prepared. I wanted to know the purpose of my life. I had to use my time wisely. I had to discover God's plan for my life. During these days, I was so confused. I used to know what my next step would be. I had goals and knew what I wanted. Now I knew nothing. I kept praying and asking God so many questions. I waited for answers.

And then we received a call from my surgeon. My spleen pathology results were in.

CHAPTER 4
Jehovah Jireh
Remon

March 2017
Monday

I don't know how Dalia had the power for anything. On Monday, she spent eight hours going from one interview to another. I didn't keep track of the actual number, but it must have been at least four interviews in that span of time.

While this was going on, I attended some of the interviews and orientations held for spouses, to ensure that we would support each other during the study program.

Around 4:00 p.m., someone came to the room and told me that my wife was in pain, and she couldn't stay.

We went back to the emergency room where they checked her again. We knew her spleen could rupture at any moment, if it hadn't already.

Thankfully, it hadn't. But the pain was there, and we still had two days before the surgery.

It was a horrible couple of days at home. I worried that her spleen could blow up at any moment. If I hugged her, it could rupture; if she bent over a certain way, it might rupture; if she carried a heavy grocery bag, it might rupture. Her life was constantly in danger because of something we could do nothing about. We just had to wait.

Wednesday

We woke up at 4:00 a.m.; it was still dark. We drove to the main hospital in downtown Orlando. They took her vitals, checked her in, and put her in a room, running an astounding number of tests.

The results were not good; her hemoglobin was so low. They could not perform surgery on her in this condition unless they gave her a blood transfusion and some intravenous iron. They would need her to stay at the hospital for almost five days to wait for the surgery and to get her to a point where they could operate.

They couldn't imagine how she was working, studying, and interviewing in such a bad state, let alone how she was functioning at all.

Our fifth-floor room was practically empty aside from the two of us—Dalia on her bed, getting infusions and medication to deal with the pain, and myself on the recliner, studying and readying myself for my own tests. I spent the entire time there until they finally got her to a state where they could perform the surgery.

Early one morning, they took her to the operating room. The operation took almost four hours. The surgeon called me to give hourly updates, but I remained worried about her. After they finished, someone called my name and took me to a small room to speak to the surgeon.

He said they had saved her life, the spleen was totally out, and she was in recovery. However, the spleen was so enlarged, and there was a disturbing number of cysts and inflammation visible. The doctor mentioned he sent some samples for pathology testing, and the results would be back soon.

For the first time, it hit me.

For the last couple of weeks, I had thought it would all be over after this surgery.

We didn't know that this would not be the end.

March 2017

After the first surgery, Dalia started her recovery. We stayed at the hospital for another ten days. The incision site hurt so much because a lot of nerves and muscles had to be cut, which took a long time to heal.

I kept telling myself that everything would pass. *She's no longer at risk of dying; Dalia will heal,*

I will pass my test, and we will be back to our normal life soon.

The doctors put her on pain medications. I continued to study beside her hospital bed. I had to get three weeks off work because there was no one else to stay with Dalia at the hospital.

I started spending from our savings, a small account to begin with. I knew our savings wouldn't last long. I needed help badly.

Finally, they discharged Dalia, and I was able to go back to work. But she had to stay home by herself all day. She could do a few things, but she definitely needed help with a lot of her normal activities.

I was so tired; Dalia was in so much pain. The splenectomy was not an easy surgery to recover from. Also, when they remove your spleen, you become less immune to disease. She had to get vaccines for pneumonia, meningitis, and hepatitis.

April 2017

At this time, they announced at the church that Dalia needed help. So, some friends helped us by preparing meals or by checking on Dalia while I was at work. But the biggest help we got was Mays. She and Dalia weren't friends at the time, but she was the one who helped Dalia almost every day when I was at work.

The second biggest help was financial. I spent three weeks off work, our savings was almost depleted, and the emergency room and bills for scans started to arrive in our mailbox. I had no idea how I would afford the rent for that month. Then someone from the church handed me some money and said, "It was gathered to help you at this rough time." I was so glad that someone thought about this. I had never mentioned to anyone the financial issues we were having. This money kept the family afloat.

I organized my work schedule and study schedule better. Dalia also started to heal, and I felt like *okay, now we can forget all about the last few weeks and live normal lives*—until Dalia's surgeon called.

He said he had good news and bad news. The good news was that he was sure that the spleen had been totally removed as well as the cysts. But the bad news was that the pathology report showed unclassified high-grade pleomorphic sarcoma—a very rare type of cancer.

High grade means it is likely to spread; pleomorphic means its origin is unidentifiable and it could arise from any part of the body; sarcoma means it's a soft tissue cancer. Two different labs confirmed the same results. The doctor advised that we should consider following up with an oncologist.

After this phone call, I couldn't even speak; l was in shock. This had turned into a nightmare, and I couldn't wake up. So many thoughts to process. *What am I to do now? I can barely keep the ship going; I don't think I can manage any further. I can't keep up with everything going on.*

I knew I had to calm down. *I have to make sure Dalia is not scared. I don't want her to feel all the troubles we have.*

I tried to convince myself and Dalia that this was good news. She had cancer, but it was totally removed. What's next is just a routine step and a necessary follow up for any cancer patient.

I immediately started to research, and what I read about Dalia's type of cancer wasn't good at all. Soon after this phone call, I booked an appointment with an oncologist. I tried to do everything so fast. I had this feeling that if I slowed down, we would lose the battle. I tried to convince myself that my wife was a cancer survivor—her tumor was rare, but it was successfully removed. *Everything will pass soon.* I don't know if it was denial or my way to keep going without thinking that I might actually lose her one day.

"For I know the plans I have for you, declares the Lord, plans for welfare and not for evil, to give you a future and a hope."
Jeremiah 29:11

CHAPTER 5

What is the Purpose of My Life? Dalia

Am I right? Am I really in God's plan or am I living my own plan? What if I die before I achieve anything?

Was my life before a waste of time? Did I fulfill the ultimate purpose God planned for my life?

Have I focused on the wrong goals? Have I missed the essential meanings of life?

What is it, oh God?

Help me. My mind cannot stop thinking of the possibilities that could happen to me.

I am drowning; help me, Lord. Show me the way. Show me the purpose of my life. Help me find Your way. Am I still alive?

I don't want to waste any more time serving my own goals—my own plans.

March 2017

We received a call from my surgeon telling us that he had sent a sample of my spleen to two different labs to examine it. The final results were all the same.

My husband and I sat in shock. We had so

many questions. The doctor advised us to see an oncologist. I looked at Remon trying to make him feel that I was not scared or worried about these results. I wanted to convince him, and myself as well, that, yes, I had cancer, but now everything is okay. Now I am saved; there is no more pain, I am no longer at risk.

I entered my room and sent these results to my friend, a doctor in Egypt, to get her opinion about the report. I was scared and crying. It seemed no one knew anything about this type of sarcoma. I didn't want to take chemotherapy. I loved my hair—my outer looks. My appearance gives me great confidence in myself. *I am not prepared to lose my hair. I refuse to be a cancer patient.* But my friend advised me to follow up with an oncologist as well.

Remon researched doctors to find a good specialist to get his opinion about my situation.

I prayed day and night. I wanted God to do something so I wouldn't have to take chemo. I explained to God how valuable my hair and my figure were for me. I told God that I would take more pain rather than losing my hair or my outer looks. While I prayed, saying these words, I felt in my heart that my words made no sense. *How am I saying that I want to live by Your vision in my life, and at the same time I am giving You too many conditions.* So, I asked Him to give me peace to calm me down and to prepare me before any other step came.

We booked an appointment with a good oncologist. When I entered the hospital, the first thing I saw was a shop on the first floor full of wigs and different types of hats. When we entered the oncologist's lobby, I looked around and saw his patients. They were so sad; their bodies looked so weak; their faces were pale. The office was dreary. I couldn't breathe. My legs shook. I prayed and told myself not to worry. *I don't belong here. I am clean. I had my tumor removed. I won't need anything from this office.*

We met the doctor. He said I wouldn't need any chemo. I would just follow up every three months with scans to make sure I am okay.

I was super happy and thankful. That was exactly what I needed to hear. What I didn't know was that my oncologist said I didn't need chemo because even chemo wouldn't help this type of cancer.

CHAPTER 6

The Four Words That Changed Everything
Remon

April 2017

After the surgeon's phone call, our whole life turned upside down. My brain refused to stop thinking. I considered every possible scenario. I did a lot of reading about this type of cancer and called many of my doctor friends to ask for advice.

They all agreed it was very rare, and that sarcoma is not an easy cancer to treat. I became more isolated and spoke less and less every day. I couldn't sleep at night. My brain would not let me rest.

Appointment day

The office was almost full. *So many people in pain battling cancer.* But the worst part—Dalia was absolutely the youngest patient in the waiting area.

We saw the oncologist; he was brief. His conclusion was that she may not need chemotherapy. But he still needed to speak with the tumor board. They would decide the best course of action.

Every cancer hospital has a tumor board. A surgeon, an oncologist, and a pharmacist. Most cancer cases are very close calls, and treatment regimen cannot be a single-doctor decision. The tumor board votes for the best recommendation depending on the survival chances and treatment benefits weighed against the risks and complications.

Chemotherapy would be a nightmare for Dalia, and since she knew that she had cancer, she was very depressed.

A few days later, the doctor called and said the tumor board voted that she didn't need chemotherapy. It was great news for us. We needed something to celebrate and ignored the fact that the tumor board decided not to do chemotherapy only because the chemotherapy is not effective with this kind of sarcoma.

July 2017

We had a quiet two months. I was finalizing my study, Dalia's wounds were healing, and the pain medications helped with her pain for a little bit.

I passed my test and became a licensed pharmacist. I had worked so hard for this moment—my dream.

I was so happy to get my license for two reasons. First, now I wouldn't have to study many hours every day. I had been exhausted for the last couple of months. Second, being a pharmacist would make us financially stable. I would be able to pay all the hospital bills that had started to arrive.

Dalia threw a great celebration for me with a cake, nice dinner, and balloons all over our apartment.

August 2017

With school and study behind me and Dalia healing, my thoughts focused on the future. *I'll try to forget everything that happened in the last few months. Now I have a great job, Dalia will feel better soon, and everything will be okay.*

However, Dalia's pain medications were not doing a good job. I thought she might need a higher dose. But that didn't make sense to me. Her surgery had been five months ago. She shouldn't need a higher dose; she should actually need a lower dose.

We booked another appointment with the oncologist; he was concerned. Worsening pain was not a good sign. She was due for her routine scan, so the doctor ordered these scans to be done ASAP.

That was her first routine scan after

surgery. This was supposed to be done every three months to follow up with the oncologist. The results were shocking to us, our denial for the past few weeks had come to an end.

The oncologist was brief as usual. *"The. Tumor. Is. Back,"* he said. "We need to operate to remove it again. This time we will consider chemotherapy for sure."

Four words, but they changed our lives for the second time. I felt we were trapped in a nightmare with no escape.

"No temptation has overtaken you that is not common to man. God is faithful, and he will not let you be tempted beyond your ability, but with the temptation he will also provide the way of escape, that you may be able to endure it."
1 Corinthians 10:13

CHAPTER 7

It's Only a Matter of Time Until... Dalia

I believe, and my beliefs come from the way the Lord Himself always treats me. I believe my Lord is all good and all merciful. He understands my feelings and appreciates every detail no matter how big or small; how significant or insignificant it is. I believe God does not keep us from temptations, but He gives us the power to fight when trials come. He loves me in every way possible. I believe that God does not tempt us with evil. Instead, He gives us peace, comfort, and sympathy in the middle of the temptation. He even gives us the strength and the preparation before it starts.

In my case, it took me five months to accept the fact that my world would not collapse if something bad happened. As I continued to pray, He worked within my heart to shape and change my thoughts and to calm my fears helping me face every new step in my path.

September 2017

The CT scan found my tumor had come back in the same spot. I was shocked; I had so many questions, but the oncologist told us that we had no options. I would need another surgery; it couldn't be put off. Until that day, I hadn't told my family or friends in Egypt that I had cancer. I didn't want them to panic; I thought we had removed the tumor and there would be no need for them to worry about something in the past. But after this news, I needed them to know. I needed their support even if they couldn't be with me physically. I needed their emotional support and their prayers.

I had not healed from the first surgery and this one would be in the same spot. I still had so much pain from the first time. But what other options did I have?

We returned to my surgeon to arrange for the second surgery. The doctor was so sad and anxious. Everything happened so fast, I had no time to even think about what was happening.

The surgery was on my left side; they cut all the muscles and the nerves for the second time. During recovery, I screamed in pain. I couldn't move; it was horrible.

A couple of days later, I was in my room when a team of oncologists came to discuss my case and the next step. I was by myself; Remon had gone home to bring something to me. They started to explain the type of cancer I had and how aggressive it was. They needed me to read about the type of chemo I could take. I was in so much pain, I couldn't remember anything they said. I didn't have the power to argue or ask any questions.

I spent a week in the hospital. After surgery, we booked an appointment with a new oncologist in the main hospital. He was part of the team I met during my second surgery.

I started to prepare myself for what I thought he would say. I needed chemo, but I didn't know that my case was more complicated than that.

The doctor told me that my cancer was so aggressive, and this type of sarcoma has no cure. "We could try chemotherapy on you," he said. "But this chemo will be aggressive. Each session will be five days, 24 hours a day. Literally, you will fall apart and for nothing. Your life expectancy is six to nine months maximum if the chemotherapy doesn't work. I will give you a strong pain medication to help you with your pain now. Until . . ."

I couldn't hear the rest of his words. I looked at Remon; he was crying like a baby. For me, I felt like I was hit by a train. *Is he talking to me?* His office was on the 11th floor in the hospital. *Why are you even bothering to tell me all this information? You could simply tell me to jump out of this window and die. What choices do I have now? He is simply telling me to choose how I will die. What should I do? Should I go to Egypt and say goodbye to my family or stay here with Remon and Hodor, my dog?*

My heart ripped in pieces.
My brain stopped.
My tears ran like a flood.

CHAPTER 8

Rage, Isolation, and Compassion
Remon

September 2017

Our world changed forever. It wasn't an isolated incident that we could forget when time passed. It was becoming the reality that we couldn't change and the fact that we couldn't deny.

Dalia's cancer was so aggressive. It came back so quickly. Most cancers take six months to one year to come back if they are extremely aggressive, but in Dalia's case, it came back in less than four months. This didn't help our chances at all.

I held so much rage inside me. I was angry at God because He allowed this to happen. I was angry at the world because we wouldn't have the chance to live a normal life. I was angry at people because all they offered were just words. Nothing was going to cure my wife.

I called her surgeon again, connected him with the oncologist, and set up an appointment for surgery. I felt like we couldn't beat this thing. Dalia had almost given up, and if I gave up too, I would lose her forever.

Déjà vu. That's what we felt the second time we went through the whole process. Home prep and antiseptic shower for surgery, waking up early, Dalia's prep in the hospital. Me. Alone in the waiting room.

Except one substantial difference—the first time we didn't know it was cancer. Then, we were saving her life, and we had hope. This time, we didn't have hope at all. It was a lost battle. There was a zero guarantee the tumor wouldn't come back and no guarantee that Dalia would be okay.

The second surgery was even more painful than the first. The surgeon had to cut through the same nerves and muscles again. This led to a more painful recovery, even worse than the first surgery. The first time, we thought that everything would be over soon; now we both knew it would not be over any time soon.

I had a mountain of emotions at this point; I felt powerless because Dalia had worse pain than before. I was angry because I knew Dalia didn't deserve any of this pain. I was frustrated—there was no hope in the near future. If her cancer came back this fast, it could come back again in the next four months.

This time, the hospital team set us up with a different oncologist. He was a facts-only guy. He gave us the bare facts in one visit. "The chemotherapy usually doesn't work in her case, but if it does work, it only extends a patient's life for a year or two."

Basically, he was telling Dalia that she should give up and keep her outer appearance, live on pain medications, and wait for her cancer to come back, or she could go on with chemotherapy with no great results expected.

I was so furious. I was angry at everything. I withdrew myself even more and stopped answering phone calls altogether. I didn't want to talk to anybody; I didn't have the power to talk or to explain myself to anyone. What could I say to people when they called to ask about Dalia? I had to repeat the same story for everyone who called. I told the story of the hospital, the scans, the surgery—to everyone. I was exhausted, physically and mentally, and needed some peace.

I had the feeling that Dalia had no motive to fight. She didn't want to take the treatment. The only thing she could think about was seeing her family before she died.

October 2017

We changed a lot; we became more depressed. Dalia was devastated. I spoke less and avoided social connections. But one thing changed in me for the better. Now I could feel the pain of my cancer patients.

I found I came to be more compassionate, and I talked to them a bit more. I tried to be more comforting, to give them more of my time. I didn't do that intentionally, but I found myself doing that almost all the time since we had an unpleasant experience with a rough doctor. This experience almost made us give up on treatment. *Until one day*.

I was talking to one of my patients. She mentioned that her husband had kidney cancer and almost lost hope because his cancer came back many times before he finally went to Moffitt Cancer Center. He had now been cancer free for four years.

Her words gave me hope for the first time in weeks. I booked an appointment for Dalia with an oncologist at Moffitt. I was really looking for the tiniest chance. This hospital was a hundred miles away from home, but I decided to get a second opinion from them.

The day before the appointment, I started to feel hopeful again, that we could get through this. I read amazing things about this hospital; I hoped for a different opinion and other options.

But I was wrong, again.

"Put on then, as God's chosen ones, holy and beloved, compassionate hearts, kindness, humility, meekness, and patience,"
Colossians 3:12

CHAPTER 9

Shopping NOT—with a New Friend Mays

Please, God, like how you healed my little son when he was one year old, I want you to heal Dalia. This is just me; my prayers are very simple, yet I knew deep inside, He would bring healing to her weak body. I never thought for a second that I would lose her. Doctors said that her chances to live were 10 percent, maybe even less. But for me, this was just another story of how God is good and how His hands are powerful.

The first time I met Dalia was in a youth group. I felt she was different from the rest of the people. The others were great, of course! But Dalia looked more like me, and we tend to like people who we find familiarity with, don't we?

She took the first step! She called me; told me she wanted to go shopping with me. I immediately agreed because I really wanted to get to know her. We planned to meet three days after. However, that shopping day never happened.

"Have you heard what happened?" the leader of the group asked me.

"No?"

"It's Dalia! She's very sick!"

"What? Why? What's wrong with her?"

"We don't know yet!"

We weren't close at that time; I didn't know if she needed space or if it was okay to call her, to ask if she was fine or not. I was worried about her, but I did nothing. Except for when they told us that Remon needed help. He needed someone to take their home keys and to take care of Dalia while he was at work. She was recovering from her first surgery. She was in much pain, home alone, and helpless. I don't even recall the whole keys incident. I didn't even know what Remon looked like, but I felt in my heart that I needed to be there, to pick up those keys. So that's what I did.

When I reached their house, there was some noise inside. I knocked, and I heard something. It was Dalia! She was screaming from her lungs.

Remon opened the door.

I panicked; I didn't understand what was wrong with her. It was like she was shouting out of pain. My heart ached at that scene; I cried when I saw her like that, however, seeing her like that moved something in my depths. I decided I would do all I could to make her feel better again.

My name is Mays; I have Arabic origins. When I first married, I lived far away from my parents' house. In that part of the city, people spoke a different language; they had a different culture, and everything was just different. As an Arab, it was hard for me to get used to this, so I just felt alone. When I was sick, I was alone! When I needed help, I was alone. When I wanted to share a happy moment, I was alone. It was tiring! But then, I found some people who made me feel better. When I saw how helpless Dalia was, I remembered those past years, and I felt it was my turn to pay it forward. It was my turn to support a person in need and make her feel good again.

I was grateful to God because I didn't have a tight schedule, and I was grateful to God because I had a very kind husband too. He would say, "Go! Be there with Dalia! She needs you; I can stay with the kids."

So, I did. I felt it was my duty to do this, especially since other women from church weren't available; most of them were very busy, so I decided to be there for her. I would stay all morning with her when Remon was at work or when he was studying for his exams, and that was when we got very close. We had our fun moments; we would just watch funny talk shows, laugh at them together, and talk for hours. We laughed at

Hodor, her dog, and at stories from the past. It was a blessing being around her, but it sometimes required strength too.

My heart broke every time I saw a surgery wound. I felt anxious when I heard bad news, and there was so much! I felt pain in the depth of my soul when I saw her suffer. Sometimes, I couldn't even show my real emotions. I couldn't show I was devastated because I didn't want her to feel more pain, so I would smile, get myself together, and talk to her, encourage her, and support her. The moment I reached my home every time, I cried myself to sleep. I lived precious moments with Dalia that were full of God's glory, but I lived some cruel moments too.

"Love is mysterious. I have never understood how it works. How someone can feel your pain even if he lives on a different continent thousands of miles away."
Dalia

CHAPTER 10

Mysterious Love, Incredible Faith
Dalia

September 2017

At this time, my youngest sister was engaged. She should have been preparing for her wedding, but instead, she postponed everything until I felt better. After we calmed a little from the bad news that chemo would not work for me, I asked Remon not to tell my family because I really wanted my sister to have her wedding. I didn't want them to be heartbroken about me.

I called Mirna, my youngest sister, to tell her that I had very good news from the doctor, that my body was fine. "I even want to come celebrate with you," I said. "So, plan a date for your wedding, and I will book my ticket. It will be awesome." I tried to convince my sister to do it within the next two months. I knew I didn't have much time left. I wanted to make sure she had her dream wedding with no sadness. She shocked me with her response. I remember her exact words.

"I will book my wedding date after I see a report from the hospital saying that your body is totally cured. I am praying for a miracle," she said, "and He promised to give it to you and everyone will know that."

I couldn't hold back my tears. I cried loudly. She made it so hard for me; I wanted her to say yes. I called her the next day. She kept insisting, so I told her everything I knew. It was very hard on her. But I realized, I needed someone to lean on, I needed her faith and prayers. I needed somebody to tell me that everything was going to be okay.

In the meantime, Remon kept searching and studying about my sarcoma. He looked for specialists in this rare type of cancer.

While he was searching, one of his customers told him about Moffitt Cancer Center in Tampa. He convinced me to go there for a second opinion.

Remon, my family, my friends in Egypt, and I were so worried and overwhelmed with all the recent bad news.

At Moffitt Cancer Center, we met with an amazing oncologist. He is still my doctor today. He said almost the same thing as the others, but in a different way—a merciful way. He said, "Your chances are very low. The chemo we will give you is horrible, different than any other one. And, if you decide to do it, you need to start as soon as possible."

Depression set in. This was not an easy

decision. Remon wanted me to try anything even if the chance was one percent. My thoughts were scattered. *If I start chemo with low chances of survival, I will not be able to travel. I could die before I see my family. And the last memory of me for Remon is my damaged, broken, hospitalized version of me. Oh, God, I need your help. Give me wisdom; enlighten me to make the right decision.*

"I loathe my life; I will give free utterance to my complaint; I will speak in the bitterness of my soul. I will say to God, Do not condemn me; let me know why you contend against me. Does it seem good to you to oppress, to despise the work of your hands and favor the designs of the wicked?"
Job 10:1-3

CHAPTER 11

Where are You, God?
Dalia

October 2017

I was so depressed and devastated. I felt that God had abandoned me. My questions had no answers.

I asked God, "Did you save me to let me die in this dreadful way? And if you want me to die, why did you not take me before I started all these horrible surgeries? I listened to you. I was ready. I accepted the idea of taking chemo—of losing my hair. Why this type of cancer? Why this type of chemo? Why do I have to suffer this much for nothing?"

I felt myself swimming in self-lament, remembering all the bad things that had already happened to me. And how life had become so hard without a break. How I didn't even have the luxury to spend my last days with my family and the people I love. I was drowning in self-pity and that was so dangerous. These words were just between God and me.

In the middle of my struggles, which I didn't share with others, some people decided to give me their opinions about my situation. And that was more frustrating than the cancer. Some told me that I was lucky because "Now God is tormenting you to purify your soul before you die." Others told me "You have to confess your sins, so He can take this penalty away from you."

I decided to resist what my mind and those people were trying to do. I worship an amazing, loving, righteous, and merciful God, not that sadistic weird one they described. I continued reading His Book refusing all the negative voices even if the voice came from my own mind. I read the book of Job. That was the perfect book for me to read. It changed my whole attitude. It gave me the strength and the understanding for what was to come and for people's reactions.

I was truly amazed when I read about Job's friends. After reading about Eliphaz, one of Job's closest friends, I posted a summary of my thoughts on my Facebook profile.

Eliphaz's character never fails to impress me. We meet this character a lot in our lives. Personally, I have had lots of encounters with this character lately. To be honest, I'm grateful to the Bible which shows us different characters, so that we don't break down when it gets too hard. I respect this character! For real! But I realize we should take care of some serious things.

A huge part of Eliphaz's pep talk was true. We hear a lot of it in worship songs and in services. We use Eliphaz's words as praise on a daily basis. What hurts me is to see that this Eliphaz is a wise man. He keeps talking about his experiences with God, which may truly be one of a kind, but then slowly, he starts to judge you. He starts to even tell you that this is God's will for you. Maybe he will let you doubt God's love! Maybe he will let you question your worth! You won't even notice it! All of this is because he's only seeing your story from his own perspective. It's funny how this perspective focuses on God's will for your own life! It's also funny that if he could understand God's will for his own life, he wouldn't be saying such things.

If you're in Job's shoes, don't listen to him. Even if the words are beautifully written. Even if they're from the scriptures. Judge the words yourself before you believe them.

And if you're Eliphaz, please consider every word you want to say. There's more to the world than your experiences and encounters. God is not limited! You will never fully understand Him. Maybe your words are correct, but maybe also, they don't suit the person you're talking to.

—My Facebook profile November 2017

CHAPTER 12

A False Hope
Remon

October 2017

We woke that morning with a lot of hope. We drove a hundred miles for a second opinion. And the feedback about this hospital was just incredible.

The moment we walked in, we felt something different about the place. The staff welcomed us; they helped us complete insurance pre-approvals, set up scans, and doctor's appointments. They also transferred Dalia's health medical records from our previous doctors.

But still, the disease is so aggressive and all the patients there were in great pain. I looked at the faces of those in the waiting area and tried to guess who might be in remission and who had already won their battle. Then I stopped. I tried to escape my fears by giving myself false hope. Then, my focus changed; I started to see the sufferings. The people looked so weak; almost all of them had lost their hair. However, there was a great difference in this waiting area. For the first time, I saw a few patients around the same age as Dalia.

We were not alone.

We had a better experience with this doctor, even though he probably said the same thing as the other oncologist. But the way this doctor said it was better for Dalia.

For me, it was a shock. I had hoped for a better option. This hospital had a great reputation for cancer patients and should have known so much more. *If they provide the same evaluation, this means we have no escape and Dalia is officially sentenced to die.*

The doctor said, "The chemo is an option, but in Dalia's case, it only extends the time she will live. When a patient is this young, Dalia must consider the treatment. Her body is better fit to fight this disease than older patients. No one can force her to do anything she doesn't want to do. She has to provide her consent for every step. At the end of the day, statistics say only 13 percent of this cancer shows complete remission with treatment."

It was a hard decision to make. I tried to convince Dalia to fight; I couldn't accept that I might lose her. But she seemed like she couldn't fight anymore. To Dalia, it was a lost cause. She either died in less than 12 months or take the treatment with an 87 percent chance that she could live for two years. During this chemo journey, the pain and suffering would be indescribable, and she would become a different person than what she used to be.

Dalia needed time to think.

CHAPTER 13

Thousands of Miles Away
Neveen

What do you do when you hear this: "Your sister is dying! Please do something." What do you do when you are thousands of miles away from that one person who needs you most? Do you cry? Do you lose hope? Or do you convince the people around you that you must go, be with her, support her, make her food, and just be under the same roof with her? In my case, I did none of these. I only prayed.

October 2017

My mom was very sick. She had to undergo several procedures, laparoscopic mainly, but still very painful. It was hectic, and she was in severe pain. The whole family was under huge pressure, but during that time, I went through a different kind of pain because while my mom needed me, my sister did too.

However, my husband, Rafik, did not want to let me go. "Neveen, it's out of the question! You cannot leave us. The kids and I need you."

I did not argue. I totally understood his

point, but my heart cried to God, asking for a miracle. Because, deep inside, I knew I was supposed to be somewhere else. Rafik was not selfish to want his wife to be at home; this I understood very well, but I still needed to be with my sister. I did not know when I would see her again; I didn't know *IF* I would ever see her again, so I continued to cry out to God. "Breathe life into her soul," I cried. "Please, God! Breathe life into her soul." These were the only words I could utter—the only words I could speak. I didn't ask for healing, and I didn't ask that she would not have to encounter chemotherapy. I only asked this: *Breathe. Life. Into. Her. Soul.*

Then one day, during these hard times, I had this phone call. I was at the hospital; we all were there with my mom. She was having one of her surgeries, and it was a tough one. I went out of the room to answer Remon's call from the U.S. He begged me to go there, to leave my family in Egypt, and be with Dalia. I did not know what to say!

"Your sister is dying . . ." Remon said.

My heart got heavier as he started to cry.

"I'll see about this," I said. I went back to my mother's room, hopeless and desperate. I found my mom screaming out in pain. I looked at her; I remembered Remon's shaking voice. I could not hold it anymore. I don't know what happened, or how it happened, but I was about to swallow my tongue!

My body reacted to my sadness! Stress overtook me; all the pressure I had tried to hide attacked me in a cruel way, making all those around me panic. My son Youssef was very quick. Before the doctors arrived, he googled my symptoms; he saved my life.

Based on Youssef's instructions, they helped me, positioned me, and I returned to normal, but on the inside, I was far from normal. I thought of what Remon had said and of what Rafik stated before; I was going through hell. My mom's screams were louder and louder, and that was when Rafik took me outside the room.

"You must go," he said.

"What? What do you mean?" I replied.

"You must go be with Dalia. Look at us here. We're all around your mom, and she's screaming out in pain. Then what about that poor soul, facing cancer, all alone?"

I remained silent. I didn't believe what I was hearing.

"Look, Neveen! If something bad happens to Dalia, I will feel guilty for the rest of my life. When I saw your mom's pain, I realized this was wrong. So, go! Be with your sister."

"I prayed that you would ask me to go," I

told him. "I didn't want to bother you with my family's issues; I couldn't tell you I needed to go."

"Darling, we're one family. Dalia is part of my family too, so go."

"And whoever gives one of these little ones even a cup of cold water because he is a disciple, truly, I say to you, he will by no means lose his reward."
Matthew 10:42

CHAPTER 14

A Cup of Cold Water
Dalia

October 2017

This verse always confuses me. Cup of cold water? Why is it a big deal? And why little ones? My thoughts were that first of all, it doesn't matter how big or small your act of kindness because all have a great impact. And second, when you do a favor for the little ones, you don't expect a favor in return. And that is exactly what happened to me.

Most of my friends are doctors, but they didn't even know what to say. My situation was so bad. When they thought about my chances medically, there was no way to survive. The chemo would be painful and wouldn't help at all. After so many discussions with Remon, my friends, and family—after nights of thinking, praying, and crying—finally, after Remon kept begging me to not give up on hope, I decided to take the chemo.

I had a call from Viva, my friend, telling me that I should prepare myself. I have now less than ten days before my first session. Maybe I should consider doing microblading for my eyebrows.

And search for a wig. And, actually, that was very good advice.

Mays and I searched for a good eyebrow place. Most of them were either bad, or they had full schedules. Finally, we found this amazing place. Mays took me there, but they told us they were fully booked for the next six months. I got so sad and told them my situation. They called the owner who was off because her husband had died a couple weeks before. They told her about me. She decided to open the place herself, just for me, on a day they were normally closed. She made me so happy. She didn't know me, but she decided to help me.

October 24 2017

A couple of days later, Mays took me to get my wig. It took us about five hours. I got tired, and Mays's kids kept calling her; they needed her back home. We bought the wig and drove home. I was so sad, so quiet. Mays was depressed seeing me like this. When we arrived, I told her to go to her kids, and I would take a nap.

When Mays left, I picked up my mirror and sat on my couch looking at my hair. I tried on the wig. I started crying and couldn't stop. For 30 minutes, my thoughts ran wild. *I hate it. I hate this. Everything is so depressing. How can I go through this? Every session will be five days. During this type of chemo, I can't move at all. I will need someone to help me all the time. Remon is depressed; he wants to stay with me at the hospital, but he has to work. Mays tries so hard to be always beside me, but her family needs her as well. The hospital is a hundred miles away from our homes. My family in Egypt are devastated, and they can't come to me. Neveen is the only one who is capable of taking care of me, and she can't leave her young boys. And my mom is sick. I am such a burden to everyone. I cannot take it anymore.* I cried hysterically.

While I was crying, Mays returned.

"Did you forget something?" I asked.

"No," she said, "I just want to hug you."

For me, that was a cup of cold water in the middle of my boiling heart. She hugged me and we both cried without saying a word. And that was all I needed.

As we cried, my dog played with the tissue box and, somehow, got his head stuck inside. He stumbled around, hitting the walls because he couldn't see anything. We watched him; it was so stupid, but hilarious. We laughed for hours. Then we took silly photos and made some crazy videos. Our moods were changed.

October 26, 2017

I kept wondering how I could care for myself when I started chemo. *How can I deal even with the tiniest details of my life? I know I will need someone beside me 24/7.*

Remon couldn't sleep thinking about how he could be there for me. He was so worried that something might happen to me while he was at work.

I give up. That's it. I cannot start this chemo. I am putting all my loved ones in a very bad situation.

Nothing in the world will make you more devastated than feeling helpless for the closest people in your life, and that's how Remon and my family felt about me. And for me, it really broke my heart giving them a very hard time like that. I couldn't stand this feeling. I decided to lift this burden from all my family and friends. I decided I would listen to the first doctor and take my pain medicine until I go in peace. I can't let anybody suffer because of me. That's my final decision.

On that same day, Mays came to visit. She was happy, well dressed, and asked me to dress up as well. It was weird. I refused, but she insisted. She told me we would take lunch outside today. I wasn't in the mood to go. Remon and Mays's kids and her husband came as well. They were smiling and happy.

I was confused. *Why do they look like that? I'm supposed to start chemo in two days. They should be worried, not smiling.*

"Our God is amazing. He cares about you more than you think. He knows you very well. You are not your circumstances. You are not a feather in the wind. Your Almighty knows what you are going through. And He cares about your every tiny little detail. He will send you the support you need at the perfect timing. Just trust Him; hang onto Him. Don't lose faith; don't lose hope. He will never let you down."
Dalia

CHAPTER 15

A Letter to Cancer
Dalia

"There she was—my beautiful little sister. She wore a white t-shirt and a short blue jacket. She was holding her dog, Hodor, and that was when I walked into the room. She saw me, and she burst into tears! She didn't know I was coming; no one told her! They preferred to let it be a surprise. On seeing me, she sobbed, and I held her tight. We hugged; I cried too, and we both couldn't believe that I was finally there. It was the answer to prayer; it was God's "Yes," and this meant the whole world."

– Neveen,

October 26, 2017

The door opened, and there she stood. I thought I was dreaming. She hugged me. I cried a lot, but this time they were tears of thankfulness. Neveen is not like any other sister. All my family depends on her. She takes care of each one of us, even our parents.

At this time, she was taking care of my mom

who had gone through many surgeries. She was also helping my youngest sister to prepare and do all the shopping for her wedding. She helped her husband in his business and studied with her boys. Mony was in middle school, and Youssef was in high school. She came from Egypt, traveled overseas, left the rest of the family for months just to be with me.

I couldn't believe it. It was impossible. But she did it; she left everything behind willing to take this pain with me. *I finally have my soul back. Finally, I can breathe again. God listens to me; He sends the perfect person for the hardest mission. I didn't ask her to come, but I need her so much.* I knew that all my family leaned on her; however, she was willing to give more than I could imagine, especially to me at this time. She was literally fighting for my life. *Her love for me is indescribable.* She knew that her presence would make a huge difference. She felt I needed her love, her help, and her companionship. She always took care of me. For her, I was not just her sister; I was her best friend.

We all went out and had dinner together. I really enjoyed that. I remember that was the last meal I could taste—the last laughter without pain—the last gathering outside without fear of infection due to my low immunity.

Hey cancer,
You may take my strength for a while,
some organs or my hair as well.
But you will never take my smile, my faith,
my hope, or my inner peace.
I am a very lucky girl. My Father is the
King of Kings.
My husband is my support.
My family spoils me with love.
My friends and my church are an army
shielding me with prayers.
For that, I will keep smiling until
the last day of my life.

I posted this before my first session of chemo.

CHAPTER 16
Side Note
Dalia

October 2017

Believe me, I am not that strong, but His presence in my life strengthens me, gives me the power and the energy to keep going. In my prayers, I always say I will not be able to do this alone. *I need You with me all the time. Strengthen me to complete my journey.*

Before I posted my letter to cancer on Facebook, I prayed all the time asking Him to enlighten me. I longed to hear His voice, to tell me what I should do. All I could feel was that He wanted me to share what was happening to me with everybody. I am not that kind of person who usually shares personal news, especially on Facebook. But His voice was so clear; He wanted everyone to know. I didn't ask Him the reason; I obeyed and shared it.

The response amazed me. My post reached many people, too many shares. I received a lot of messages from all over the world. People whom I didn't know sent me their prayers with different accents and different languages. Sometimes all I could understand was just my name and that was more than enough to lift my soul—to encourage me. Isn't that amazing? People from different countries, colors, and languages can be united when we have God's love in our hearts. We can pray, asking for healing for someone and all we know about that person is just the name and the prayer request.

What really hit me at that time was getting messages from people I knew telling me that they had cancer too. They felt they couldn't tell anyone because some of them have had a very bad experience. Close friends and family have judged them after learning about their cancer. When they saw my post, they decided to share their struggle with me. They saw me as the only one who could feel their pain. They told me then how my post gave them hope and encouragement. They even asked me to pray for them.

I realized how the world we live in is so cruel; how life is so painful and tough. Your friend, neighbor, or even relative can die in silence and you wouldn't even know. Be compassionate; you don't know what kind of conflict a person might be going through.

CHAPTER 17
A Lost Game
Remon

October 2017

There is nothing I can do to convince her to undergo treatment. Any pressure from my side will be pure selfishness. She is the one who will have to endure the pain. I know there is no guarantee. And the only thing that is certain is that she will lose her beauty, will become so weak, and her immune system will be compromised and vulnerable to any infection.

But she surprised me. One day, she finally made her decision. I knew she was doing this for me. But the other option was for us to give up, and I would definitely lose her.

A lot of preparations had to be done. She set herself to face the inevitable.

On my side, I had to find a way to help Dalia during treatment because I had to work long shifts. I called Dalia's sister, Neveen, and asked her if she could come help us during the treatment to take care of Dalia. I gave her the facts and the whole dark picture of what we had been living through and what was to come.

She wanted to surprise Dalia, so we didn't tell her. I felt Dalia needed this surprise right before starting treatment. She needed some hope and family warmth. One of her biggest fears was that she would be alone and might never see her family again.

We had to get ready for the treatment. It was not going to be easy at all. Because of my knowledge in pharmacology, I knew all the medications that the doctors gave her—the benefits and the dangers. The doctors gave her a combo. First, they gave her ifosfamide, which is extremely toxic. They added Mesna to prevent bladder bleeding, which is a direct side effect of ifosfamide. Second, they gave her doxorubicin, which is also cardiotoxic. Even if she recovered from cancer, these drugs could cause permanent damage to her heart and her body.

The hospital was a hundred miles from our home. Each treatment session would take five days, not like the normal two-hour treatment sessions that most cancer patients usually get. In her case, she had to be hooked up to the IV treatment 24/7 for five days.

The doctor educated her about the side effects and told her to expect pain, which made Dalia not so eager to start the treatment. But she was doing it for us.

Before the treatment day, I asked her oncologist to order one more scan to have a baseline image to compare with after-treatment images. Dalia had stomach pain with vomiting, so they also ordered an upper endoscopy.

She needed a port installed before she was hooked up to the chemo, and this was another surgery she had to go through. Then, they had to have a baseline evaluation of her heart, so they ordered an EKG and heart ultrasound. This enabled them to evaluate if they needed to stop the treatment at any point if her heart started to deteriorate quickly.

The hospital case organizer did a miracle by arranging all these appointments on the same day. We couldn't drive 200 miles back and forth each day to have these tests and procedures done in separate days. But one thing we hadn't considered was that all these things had to be done in one day. Dalia would have a 12-hour busy schedule with no food to get all this done.

She was exhausted, just out of a major surgery the month before, and then shuffled from one procedure to another. I felt she was fighting already even before she started chemo.

The treatment day finally came; the day we had all tried to avoid was finally here.

Dalia was to be admitted and start her treatment on the same day. We had to meet with the oncologist first to review the results of her scans and scope.

He appeared to be frustrated and sad. "Her cancer is back. Three recurrences in less than one year. Unheard of," he said. "The surgery is not on the table at all. For now, at least. We can't keep operating on you. While your cancer keeps coming back, our only hope at this moment is chemotherapy."

Hearing that, I knew we had no hope at all. Every doctor had said that chemotherapy would not have great results with this kind of sarcoma. And with this last recurrence, it was a lost game. Cancer kept scoring points, and we had no idea what to do or how to get back in the game.

"In all their affliction he was afflicted, and the angel of his presence saved them; in his love and in his pity he redeemed them; he lifted them up and carried them all the days of old."

Isaiah 63:9

CHAPTER 18
What Could be Worse?
Dalia

October 28, 2017

It was a long, exhausting day. I had to be there at 4:00 a.m. to start with the upper endoscopy, so we left home at 1:30 that morning to be there on time.

When I got there, they gave me a gown and prepared me by rubbing my whole body with alcohol tissues. I had the endoscopy at 6:00 a.m. Then they woke me and made me change to another hospital gown and rubbed my body with alcohol again to get ready for the second procedure. I was freezing. I had to fast until I finished everything.

In the first procedure, I had full anesthesia, but when it was time for my port installation, the anesthesiologist didn't want me to have another full anesthesia on the same day, so they only used a local one.

He told me not to move at all, even if I felt pain. I felt everything from the first touch of the scalpel on my cold skin, to placing the dual port inside my body, to closing the incision. I was so quiet; I didn't move. The surgeon talked to me, but at this moment, I could only hear the sound of my tears hitting my pillow. No one else could hear it, only me.

We finished at 1:00 p.m., then they started to prepare me for the CT scan. They moved me to another room. I hadn't eaten anything and started to get dizzy. The alcohol smell was killing me. They gave me four big cups full of contrast liquid that tasted awful. I had to drink it all before I could be scanned.

I tried my best to drink it, but I couldn't. Remon told me, "Push yourself a little more. We need to get everything done today. We don't have time."

At this moment, I cried nonstop loudly. I couldn't say a word or explain anything. I felt so miserable. "Stop pushing me," I said. "I have had enough today."

Remon apologized to me. I saw in his eyes how depressed, anxious, sad, and devastated he was. "If I could take it for you," he said, "I would do it without thinking."

I apologized to him. "I understand your pain and your worries. I will try again for you."

It took me more than two hours to finish the four cups. I had the scan. It was after 6:00 p.m. when we left the hospital. I ate my first meal at 7:00

that night. I was in pain. After I had finished my meal, I vomited.

We spent this night at a hotel near my hospital. My sister found blood all over my neck and my hair. She spent so much time trying to clean me because I was told not to shower after having this procedure.

Remon insisted that I should have another CT scan before I started the first chemo session. The doctors argued with him that I just had a surgery in less than six weeks and they removed the tumor. There was no way I would have another tumor in that short time.

In less than 24 hours, we learned they were mistaken.

The next day we went to the hospital to start the first chemo session. My heart beat so fast; my legs shook. I tried to encourage myself. I didn't want Neveen and Remon to notice my fears. They told us that my oncologist wanted to meet with me and Remon before I started the chemo.

When we met him in his office, he looked so sad. "I am so sorry," he said, "but there is bad news."

I thought—*What could be worse than our current situation?*

I couldn't process all that he said—I could

hear but a few words. "Your tumor. is. back."

I thought I heard him say this. *Was I right? Or was this just a nightmare?*

"In less than six weeks." He went on. "No change in our plan."

But what plan? What do you mean?

"We have no other option. You have to start chemo today." And then he finally stopped talking.

He paused to wait for us to respond. The room was so quiet. I looked at Remon; I was so worried about him. He always had words to say, questions to ask, thoughts to negotiate. This time, he was quiet. I could hear his heartbeats and his shaky breath. After this news, we both knew we had no way out. We felt that the last hope, the last ray of light, had faded away.

"What we would here and now call our happiness is not the end God chiefly has in view: but when we are such as he can love without impediment, we shall in fact be happy."
C.S. Lewis

"Do not be conformed to this world, but be transformed by the renewal of your mind, that by testing you may discern what is the will of God, what is good and acceptable and perfect."
Romans 12:2

CHAPTER 19

A New Way of Thinking
Dalia

I tell you: I served You today.
You tell me: And I will serve you every day.
I tell you: I listened to those wounded souls.
You tell me: I'm here to hear you and heal you.
I tell you: I have a heart for your children. I think
about them a lot.
You tell me: I count your heartbeats. I think of you
nonstop.
I tell you: I'm interested in that person's life.
You tell me: You're my only interest.
I tell you: I hope people accept this ministry I do.
You tell me: You don't need a ministry to be
accepted by me.
I tell you: I want to do meaningful things for you.
You tell me: You already mean a lot to me.
I tell you: I love you!
*You tell me: I walked to death for **You**, and that's*
*how much I love **You**.*

      I was 24 years old when I wrote these words to God in my diary in March 2012. On that day, God's voice was so obvious to me. I heard it so clearly; I even wrote it down. But the dilemma was that I didn't really perceive the meaning at that time.

I am a person who likes to achieve things. I set goals and care about time. I had a lot of plans, but my pain stopped everything. I prayed to God. *I don't want to waste my pain; I don't want to waste my time. I applied for this master's degree to offer and serve You more. I need to do more for You.*

But for the first time in my life, I realized that all He wanted was for me to do nothing. All He wanted from me was to calm down, rest, and enjoy receiving His love—to accept, love, and see myself the way He sees me.

I am called to have His heart, and only at this time, I will find myself involuntarily serving and sacrificing without effort. In my simplistic actions, I will reveal his unconditional love to the world.

But, love and pain; is it possible to have these two words in the same sentence? I am not a theologian. The only thing I know is what I humbly experienced through my journey with pain. Whatever the reason for your pain, He willingly chooses to bear this pain with you, to help, support, and reveal His true love for you. He does this, to shape and change your wrong image of Him and yourself as well; to be the amazing person He will enjoy in His company.

It took me years to understand who I am and who my Father is. And because He is a good Father, He cares a lot. He will never give up on me; He is so patient to wait this long for me to finally understand.

I started to fully trust Him, to finally let go of the things that once gave me fake security, to gain love and strength.

He used my pain to fix the wrong concept I had about Him and even about myself.

God Himself experienced pain for you. "For because he himself has suffered when tempted, he is able to help those who are being tempted" *(Hebrews 2:18)*. Jesus chose the cross as a physical way to express his love for you. The pain He had to go through on the cross reflects how much He was willing to suffer for us. Because Jesus united with humanity in bearing pain, you can trust that He feels your pain when you call Him. He is not distant from us. Instead, He is the only one who can understand your agony. He experienced pain emotionally and physically. For that, you can trust Him because He himself suffered to be able to help you. He walks with you step-by-step to support, love, and heal you.

My brother always says, "Pain is the greatest expression of God's love for humanity. The more you love the people, the more you will experience pain. We live in an evil world. One way or another, people suffer. The more you have God's compassionate and merciful loving heart, the more you will feel and unite with their pain." He adds, "You will look at them through His eyes and at this moment, you will understand how much God feels when you have pain, attempting to fix the distortions caused by this fallen world."

"I am weary with my moaning; every night I flood my bed with tears; I drench my couch with my weeping."
Psalm 6:6

"Give ear to my words, O Lord; consider my groaning. Give attention to the sound of my cry, my King and my God, for to you do I pray."
Psalm 5:1-2

CHAPTER 20

The Ugly Face of Cancer
Dalia

Oh cancer, oh cancer.
Oh, stupid ugly face. How many hearts do you
break?
How many lives do you take?
How much pain do you let people suffer?
How much I hate you!
I wish I had a magic wand, to eliminate you from
the roots, to stop you from harming more families.

November 1, 2017

I walked to my torment room. Changed my clothes and laid on the bed. The nurses came to hook up my port to the infusions. They tried to peel off the bands of the port, but it was sticky, and my incision was fresh and swollen. It was so painful. They took turns removing it, but my skin started to come off with the bandage.

They freaked out. "When did you have this port put in?" one nurse asked.

"Yesterday," I answered.

"That's impossible," she said. "You should have this procedure at least a week before you start chemo. We will call your doctor."

They came back five minutes later. "Your doctor said that you couldn't drive back and forth because of your husband's schedule; we have to start now." They tried again and again, but they couldn't do it.

I cried out in pain; my scar was so tender. I could see part of my flesh coming off with the bandage.

The nurses were shaking. My sister kept crying. They asked her to leave the room.

Personally, I felt pity for them and for me as well, so I decided to take it off myself. I held my skin with my hand, and with the other hand, I peeled it off slowly. Still, some parts of my skin had peeled with the bandages, but I had no choice. I had no time to spare.

I couldn't hold my tears; I was in severe pain. I had a dual port because I would take more than one type of chemo plus other infusions in each session. They installed two big needles inside my port, and then locked them in with something like a clip. When they did that, I heard my freshly-wounded flesh. A line of blood ran around my neck. Everything was so painful. My tears blended with my blood.

I had to be careful with every move; my scar was so fragile, and it was hooked to this huge infusion machine containing more than nine bags of chemo and other medicines plus saline for hydration. I would have it all for 24 hours for five days.

Then the poison started to run inside my body. I was so scared. I had read a lot about this chemo. But this torment was much more than I ever imagined. I was literally burning my life inside out.

God, if there is hell, I think it will be much more merciful than what I feel now.

I started to have heartburn; it was so bad—indescribable—with nausea and vomiting. I couldn't move or eat. It was horrible. I had all these infusions running into my body. I had to go to the bathroom almost every 15 minutes. To get up from the bed, unplug the machine, walk it with me while holding the tubes in my hand was very painful. It pulled my skin. It was so huge; I couldn't close the bathroom door. And yes, it was only three footsteps from my bed to the bathroom, but for me, it felt like passing the Pacific Ocean.

My eyes kept staring at the clock on the wall in front of me. It felt like the clock wasn't working. With the pain from the needles, my vomiting, and crying, it felt like eight hours, and only five minutes had passed. Time stood still.

My skin loosened and became darker.

Finally, four days passed; I couldn't stand any more. *Just one more day, and I will go home and be strong again.* At that moment, something felt wrong with my tongue and mouth. I couldn't control it. My tongue and gums swelled and turned white.

Remon looked at me and freaked out. "Dalia, stop doing that. You're scaring me."

I couldn't explain it. I felt terrible pain; my lower jaw felt as though it had broken; it went the other direction.

Remon called the nurse. In less than a minute, my room was filled with doctors and nurses. They unhooked all the lines stopping the chemo and gave me other medications in hopes of resolving my problem.

The next day, they continued the chemo session. Instead of staying five days, it lasted for seven days. I was so quiet; my tears ran the whole time. I wanted to scream, but I didn't want to put Remon and Neveen in more pain.

Finally, I finished the first session and left the hospital. Even though I was still in so much pain, it was a very happy moment for me to go home, stop this horrible medicine, see my friend Mays and Hodor, my dog. I was so thankful just for leaving.

Mays greeted me at home with a very nice

meal, but the heartburn was so bad, I couldn't eat. My sister gave me some fruit. It tasted so good; however, I found out later that fresh fruit was the worst thing to eat because it might lead to infection.

Neveen looked at me. "I am happy you didn't lose your hair."

"It will fall out soon," I said, "but don't worry, dear, I am prepared for that."

She helped me to my bed. "I will put your phone on your nightstand," she said. "Call me if you need anything."

All my body hurt. I felt this voice inside me say, "You will die today." As much as I dreamed for all this pain to end, I refused to give up. I called my sister who took my temperature. It was very high. She woke Remon at 3:00 a.m.

He called my oncologist.

"Take her to the nearest hospital. She needs to get medical attention ASAP; she might have developed an infection." **Then my doctor** called the hospital to tell them my situation and what they had to do with me and how important it was for them to be quick.

My pain was beyond anything I could imagine. This was the first hospital I had gone to. They hooked up infusions for me and did some tests. My immunity was zero, so they moved me to a special sterile room.

In my heart, I talked to God. *Please give me strength. My pain is so bad. Every cell in my body screams out.* Even the bed hurt. It didn't have a mattress because it might contain bacteria, and I had nothing to fight off an infection. All my body swelled, even my tongue. Too many needles. Even in my stomach. My lymph nodes started to swell; I had a huge one under my arm. I screamed out in pain; I couldn't lift my arm. Everyone freaked out thinking it was another tumor. They sent me for another CT scan.

I couldn't lift my arm for the scan, so the nurses tied my arms up together until the scan was finished. I cried and screamed in pain until they put my arm down. Thank goodness it wasn't another tumor.

I was there for three days; I really needed to go home. I hated everything around me. Every smell made me want to vomit. All I needed was some warm homemade soup. While I was thinking about soup, Mays delivered a bowl of soup to the hospital for me and a nice dinner for Neveen and Remon. I never in my life thought that a bowl of soup would make me that happy, thankful, and grateful.

CHAPTER 21
"Does Chemotherapy Cause Death?"
Neveen

November 2017

On my second day in the U.S., I had to face the fact that my sister would undergo two procedures and multiple tests and scans in one day.

That night in the hotel room, I looked at my sister's body; I looked at her neck and her hair, and noticed they were covered in blood. I took her to the bathroom to wash off the blood; her own blood. *How much did she bleed?* I kept the thought to myself. And I combed her hair; it was long, and it was beautiful, and I was angry! I was angry because I knew what would happen later to that beautiful hair. I tried to fight the thoughts and sleep them off.

The next day, we went back to the hospital. Remon and Dalia had to see the oncologist before starting chemo; he had bad news.

Suddenly, we were not just preventing the tumor from coming back; instead, we were fighting a recurrence that was hungry for my sister's soul, again. It didn't make sense! And it was unfair.

During the first session, Dalia had a terrible

reaction; I saw death. It was one of the worst days in my whole life. It destroyed me on the inside. My sister nearly died in front of me, but God decided it was not her time yet.

I couldn't sleep at all. I lost my appetite; I only had a quarter meal a day. We were not allowed to use Dalia's restroom because it was contaminated with chemo. I had to walk a very long corridor in order to use a different toilet. It wasn't so bad though because I used this time to pour out my soul. I cried. I cried and I prayed. It was hard, and I was weak, but I had to be strong for her! I would wipe my tears away, and go back to the room to fight this battle with my little sister.

Seven days passed; it was time to finally leave the hospital. What a relief it was to be back home. Dalia was having a hard time getting back her appetite. But on that day, she craved fruit. I remember how her face lit up when she saw the plate. I cut the fruit neatly and decorated the plate. It looked so adorable. She loved it, and she asked for more. I was happy to make her another one before she went to bed. However, that night, something bad happened.

After finally sleeping, she felt she had a fever, so she called me. When I checked her temperature, we were sure something was wrong. I woke Remon as quickly as possible, remembering

Dalia's question to her doctor.

"Does chemotherapy cause death?" she asked him.

The answer. "It usually does not, but those who have died had an infection and fever before."

My heart was racing, and Remon called Dalia's doctor to ask him what to do.

We went to a hospital that was ten minutes away from home. The same night that we celebrated Dalia finally coming back home was a night we spent in a hospital, only a different one, because Moffitt was far away. It was tough. It was really tough, but we were tougher. We had to be tougher—in order to survive.

CHAPTER 22

Why Doesn't the Clock Move?
Remon

November 2017

During the first chemo session, I took a week off from work to be with Dalia at the hospital. I pushed her to get the treatment; I saw it as our only option. But I never imagined that the treatment could be so bad. From the first hour, as soon as they hooked Dalia to the machine, she started to change—as they injected *poison* into her body.

Food was tasteless to her; she had no appetite and experienced constant, terrible heartburn. She couldn't move at all, even to go to the bathroom. All the time, she had her eyes fixed toward the clock on the wall, waiting for time to pass. Time moved so slowly, and the nights were endless.

I tried to cheer her up by turning on TV, but she couldn't watch anything.

The nurse suggested that she take a walk around the wing. We tried that a couple of times, but soon she had no power to do it anymore.

The doctors worried about possible

reactions to the treatment. One day, while I was talking to her, she started to do strange things with her mouth. I said, "Dalia, this is not funny. Stop."

She tried to stop, but she couldn't. There was something wrong with her mouth. I freaked out and called the doctor.

The doctors didn't know what was happening. They thought it was a reaction to one of the medications. They couldn't decide which one, since they were injecting her with so many meds at the same time.

They stopped the treatment until they could resolve this issue. *Oh, my poor Dalia*, I said to myself. She spent her time watching the clock, counting seconds, waiting for this to be over, and now treatment was halted, and we had to stay extra days. We had no idea how long.

After stopping treatment for one day, they decided to continue and challenge the reaction again. Thank, God! It was only a 24-hour delay. When they hooked up the medicines the next day, nothing happened, so after seven days, they discharged Dalia.

They sent her home with lots of instructions. "Drink lots of water, and fill this prescription for Neulasta injections." They warned her to be careful of any kind of infection because her white blood cell count was so low and her body would be vulnerable to any infection. But we were both so happy to be home.

The first injection was to be administered 24 hours after discharge. This shot would stimulate her body to produce white blood cells. After three or four days, they told us her white blood cell count would go up to a safe level. During the first few days after discharge, we would have to watch for any symptoms of infection, mainly fever, even the mild elevation we had to report to the doctors.

That night, Dalia's temperature went to 101. I was sleeping in a separate room trying to get some rest because I had to work in the morning. Neveen woke me up. I called the doctor.

He said, "Take her to the closest emergency room—immediately."

There, they put her in an isolation room. No one went in without a mask or gloves. Dalia's contact with others was at a minimum. It was almost a quarantine.

We had only been home for 24 hours; we couldn't even rest from the one-week marathon we just had at the first chemo session. They gave her lots of antibiotics, ran many cultures to determine the infection type, and did lab work every day to keep track of her white blood cell count.

Her bones ached; she couldn't rest at all. The main side effect of the Neulasta injections is bone ache, as this shot stimulates her bone marrow to produce white blood cells.

Dalia said, "I feel something is crushing my bone into powder." She cried and asked them to send her home; she needed a break.

And to be truthful, we all did.

Finally, after three days, they sent us home. Dalia longed for rest. You can't really sleep in a hospital.

This time, we stayed home for almost ten days, and before we knew it, it was time for her second chemo session. It was time to repeat this all over again.

"Behold, God is my helper; the Lord is the upholder of my life."
Psalm 54:4

CHAPTER 23

What Matters to God is
What We are Willing to Give
Dalia

November 13, 2017

I started to recognize that parts of my skin, nails, and hair started to fall off.

My hair fell everywhere I went. It made me so sad. But in my mind, I said to myself, *I am not going to let that hurt me.*

When we got home, I decided to shave my hair off. I couldn't do it by myself because I still couldn't lift my arms or even move.

I called Mays and asked her to help me with this. She came right away and sat beside me. She tried to convince me to just cut my hair shorter, not to totally shave it. She cried and begged me to do it that way. I didn't have the energy to negotiate with her. She was so depressed. I tried to explain to her, but she kept insisting not to shave it, but just make it shorter.

She left me no other choice. "Look at me!" I said. I grabbed a lock of my bangs with my fingers, and it came right off. She was startled and cried loudly. I tried to calm her down. "I am fine with cutting off my hair." I was not fine on the inside. I felt rage and mixed feelings. I was sad and frustrated, all at the same time, but so strong and decisive.

She finally stopped crying and agreed to help me shave it. We all were so quiet; all you could hear at this moment was the sound of the scissors cutting my hair, then the machine shaving the rest. It was so stressful to all of us; it felt like the time suddenly moved in slow motion. Pain and sadness surrounded us. I could feel Mays's tears falling on my shoulders. I held in my tears. I didn't want to make it harder for Mays.

I closed my eyes and talked to God. *Give me the strength; help me, God. My hair is precious to me, but I still believe You are good. I believe in Your righteousness. I know You will compensate and bless me. One day these dark days will end.* At this moment, I had a calming peace in my heart. That was beyond my own strength; that was God himself hugging my poor soul.

Then Remon asked Mays to shave off his hair.

After we finished, Mays went home. Before she left, I noticed her face and all her body turned red. Mays has a condition, when she becomes scared, depressed, or under a lot of stress, her body reacts this way. I was so worried about her.

I put a cotton turban on my head because I felt shy to let Neveen and Remon see me bald.

Remon came and hugged me. "You don't have to wear this," he said. "I love you and I see you as so beautiful all the time. I need you to be comfortable. All I need from you is to survive."

That felt so good in the middle of this chaos.

After we calmed down, I asked Neveen and Remon to help me go to Mays's home. I needed to let her know that I was fine. We visited them, watched a movie together, and had some laughs. Then we went back home.

I was in so much pain the whole time. My body hurt so much. Nothing was easy, even breathing was difficult. I couldn't even take in a breath; my mouth was swollen. My teeth ached so much. It was total agony.

CHAPTER 24

Are They Supportive Like They Assume?
Mays

November 2017

People are just different from one another. This is something that I have learned. Some will cry; some will claim that it's a lie. "The doctors are lying! It's not cancer; they just want the insurance money." Some will try to find a spiritual cause to what's happening. I met all these kinds of people during that painful time with Dalia. I even met those people who would tell me, "The Lord disciplines the one He loves." I was silent most of the time. I smiled and said, "Amen." However, I had one question in my head, "Why, God? She's very young! Why let this happen to her?"

While people tried to justify what was happening—while they were explaining the "discipline" concept—I was dying on the inside. I needed my friend to be fine, and I needed all of this to end. I realized that people's reactions were not the same; those people had their own lives, their own problems, and their own business to take care of. I learned that it was okay to have those who care so much and those who don't care at all; so, it was just fine.

It was fine to go through this knowing that God was on my side, that my husband was there for me. It was fine to stick to faith and believe in a better tomorrow, and it was fine to wait for the miracle. The path was full of obstacles; sometimes it was hard to continue, but I'm grateful for the power I got from God that helped me do what I was supposed to do, however tough it was.

On one night, after Dalia's first chemo session, I went to her house. The night was hectic just like all the previous nights since the nightmare started. It was nothing new to us, but I never thought it would get any tougher. Then there it was—that moment I could never erase from my memory and that moment that still haunts me in my sleep until this day. You may find it easy; you may consider I am overreacting, but I would never be able to explain how painful this was to me.

"Mays, I want you to shave my head," Dalia said.

"What? Why? It looks nice! I thought it would just fall off after the first session, but look at that pretty hair! I think we should just leave it like that," I replied.

"Umm. No! I need you to shave my head,

please," she said.

"No."

"Please."

"No! Your hair is very important to you. I can't. I can't do this. Don't ask me to do this."

"Then look!" She grabbed a part of her hair, and it all came out in her hands. I was silent, shocked, sad, and uncomfortable with what was coming. My heart split in two. *She loves her hair. How many times has she pleaded with God not to let her hair fall? And now it's falling. How can she ask me to shave her head?*

If only she had known! If only she had known how I secretly hoped God would just surprise her; He would keep her hair on her head—just like that. If only she had known I even prayed for that, maybe then she wouldn't have requested this of me.

"Please!" she begged.

I looked at Neveen; I looked back at Dalia, at Remon—everyone, and then stress overtook me. My skin suddenly broke out with red spots; it was a condition! Something that happens to me when I am too sad, and I was too sad at that moment.

I thought about it. *If I refuse, she will have to do it herself, and she is too exhausted! She can't even raise her hands. If I refuse, she will have to go to a hair salon, where she might catch an infection. I also don't know if she can take this emotionally; perhaps, she would be ashamed, and perhaps, this would make it even harder for her. I can't let that happen.*

"All right. I will do it." And I did.

I took the shaver, and I started to talk to her. Oh, God! I showed all the strength in the world.

"It will be long again! Who knows? Maybe it will grow to be more beautiful." I smiled. "And it's gonna be okay!" I assured her—and myself.

But I knew I wasn't okay; I knew that I needed to cry out loud. In solidarity with Dalia, Remon wanted to shave his head too, and on that night, I shaved the heads of both my close friend and her partner. I shaved the heads of a cancer patient and her suffering husband—the two people living the worst days of their lives, and so this, too, became one of the worst days in my whole life.

CHAPTER 25

It's Not A Solo Journey
Dalia

November 2017

Neveen's phone rang continuously. All my friends and family from Egypt were calling her asking about me. Except my youngest sister, Mirna. After she knew the news, she stopped calling. She was so depressed and locked herself inside her room; she refused to eat or talk to anyone.

I decided to call her; I didn't have the strength to talk, but I felt that this was so important. My little sister didn't have the option to walk away or hide from this pain. I called and asked her, "Why do you keep hiding from me?"

"I . . ." she stuttered. I heard a long shivering sigh. Then she spoke with an enraged crying voice. "I am so mad, super angry at God. I prayed not to let the cancer come back. And it hit you again, not once, but twice. I prayed not to let you get chemo. And now, you are not getting just a regular chemo, but you had the worst type. I prayed not to let you lose your hair, and you lost it from the first session. I am so mad at Him, and I don't want to pray for anything ever again."

I listened carefully to her. Then I answered, "Mirna, I am fine with everything, really. My question for you now is: do you think that your prayers and requests are the things I need? Is that God's plan for me? Are your requests working with God's will for my life? I was prepared, and I accepted to walk this journey. Maybe I don't know why, but until that day comes, just help me not to lose my faith." I added, "Keep holding onto Him, doing His will, not mine. Keep reading the Bible; keep praying for me. That's the only way you can help me. I am praying for healing. I am praying for this pain to end, but I want His way, not mine. I believe in His mercy, and I know that He loves me more than anybody on earth, more than even you, my love, and I am in safe hands."

She calmed down and stopped crying. "I know I was wrong thinking that way of God. I promise to change my attitude toward prayer."

I never imagined that I would be so courageous, peaceful, and calming for my little sister during this storm.

The next day, I found her posting these words to me on her Facebook.

"It was yesterday when I saw something new. All the past weeks, I was trying so hard to keep distance from you, for us not to end up crying together like old days. Your words for me were a life lesson.

I have learned what it means when someone stands and fights.

I have learned that in the midst of pain, someone can still be thankful and grateful.

I have learned that someone can still see through faith, not through reality.

You're always the joy of our house and the cure to our souls.

You're able to shine bright despite all the circumstances.

I thank God for you, every moment.

How lucky I am to have you! You're not just a sister; you're an indescribable being!

Thank you for giving me the needed energy to go on.

Thank you for showing me something that I couldn't see on my own.

Thank you for being there for me.

I love you."

- Mirna

At this moment, I realized that God may not be working just with me in this journey. He was working with everyone around me.

When you pray, you discover not only yourself and God but also your neighbor. For in prayer, you profess not only that people are people and God is God, but also that your neighbor is your sister or brother living alongside you. For the same conversation that brings you to the painful acknowledgment of your wounded human nature also brings you to the joyful recognition that you are not alone, but that being human means being together.

Henri J. M. Nouwen
With Open Hands

"The Lord God has given me the tongue of those who are taught, that I may know how to sustain with a word him who is weary. Morning by morning he awakens; he awakens my ear to hear as those who are taught."

Isaiah 50:4

CHAPTER 26

Their So-Called Truth vs Mine
Dalia

A couple of days before I started the second chemo session, I received a message from friends who live nearby me. We used to be so close until my second surgery. They stopped visiting, calling, or even texting. In this message, they told me, "We love you, and we are praying for you."

Then some other friends visited me. They told me that I should accept God's discipline. And if I did something wrong, I need to repent, confess it, and ask for forgiveness. They said they were praying for me to have mercy from the Almighty. They kept defending God that He is righteous and good. He never does anything bad, and if something bad happened, that was all on me!

Through all my pain, I tried to maintain my stability, until that day. I was enraged. I didn't cry when I got my hair shaved, but after they had left, I cried loudly.

I wondered *Do you even know God at all? How do you judge others? And, when you say you are praying for me, do you understand what praying even means? Is it just meaningless words you say out of duty? Opinions you store in your minds and repeat without thinking? Does it have any deeper meaning for you?*

I always felt that praying is an essential way to express your love to God and the people you care about. How could the love from these people reach me in any way?

When you love your neighbor as yourself, you feel their pain. You scream to the heavens asking for mercy for your friend's misery. You pray for them day and night; you carry their pain. You ask God *why is this happening*? You ask Him for wisdom and the tongue to encourage those who might be tempted to give up hope. Without feeling tired of praying or giving up, no matter how long it takes. Because you put your full self in your friend's place. You will never have this heart until you personally meet God. He is the only one who can create this lovable and merciful heart inside you.

I remember the day when I asked my brother, Magued, about the meaning of prayers.

"Praying is when I unite with the person in their problem to the point that I can feel their pain or stress," he said. "Then I pray for God to lift this burden up from both of us. And when you reach this stage of understanding the concept of praying, you will be willing to do whatever it takes to help this person."

I was amazed by these words. And my next question to Magued was, "Do you feel my pain?"

He answered with a voice full of tears mingled with love. "I asked the Almighty to make me feel what you are going through. I want to pray for the things that you didn't even share with us. I want to stand up for you in this war. You are not alone in this. And, yes, my sister, I feel your pain."

At this moment, I realized the difference. *He is not just loving me as a brother. He has the heart of God; his love is the definition of the verse "You shall love your neighbor as yourself"* **(Matthew 22: 39)**.

Then I asked him again, "Why do people never change? Why do they have these wrong ideas and opinions about others who are in pain? Why do they walk away from me? And why do they blame me for my suffering?"

He answered, "Dear sister, don't be sad or angry. You have to feel compassion, and pity their souls. People are afraid to face pain. They will try to escape, hide, walk away if they have the chance to do that. People usually have negative thoughts about pain; no one can see any good in it.

"They prefer to hold preconceived ideas that God never lets any harm happen to the ones who worship Him. They continue doing all the religious rituals, rather than praying, searching, and asking God that they might be open to learn new lessons through this experience.

"True love is to open your heart and your mind for understanding. Walking this path without fears, asking God to help us both, and to enlighten our souls. To get to know Him even more and to survive."

"What is my strength, that I should wait? And what is my end, that I should be patient? Is my strength the strength of stones, or is my flesh bronze? Have I any help in me, when resource is driven from me?"
Job 6:11-13

CHAPTER 27

The Peak of Pain
Dalia

November 21, 2017

It was my second chemo session. This time, I knew this type of pain. I began this session with zero energy. My body was damaged. My outer appearance was totally different. I prayed for God to help me, to give me the strength to finish this one. Another torturing five days to go. From the first hour, the indescribable tormenting pain crushed my body. The rest of my nails started to fall off. Anything I touched made me bleed. My sister wrapped my finger tips to avoid the pain that came from even touching the sheets.

The hospital was freezing; my sister was wearing a wool coat. But for me, my body was burning. I couldn't even stand my clothes. I couldn't eat anything. I asked the nurses not to bring any food to my room. Every smell made me sick. The heartburn became more painful every day. If I opened my mouth, you could see vapor come out. My gums and tongue grew bigger and bigger until my teeth made scars on the sides of my tongue. I had to swish my mouth with a disgusting mouthwash all the time, or I could lose my teeth.

So many injections all over my body, too many medications for me to swallow. My body burned. I stared at the clock counting every single second. I wanted to scream, but I couldn't. I didn't want to make Neveen and Remon feel more pressure. I was powerless; I didn't have the energy to even cry.

After three days, Remon had to return to work. He called me the next day and begged me to eat anything.

I told him, "If you bring me fajitas from my favorite restaurant, which was a hundred miles away from the hospital, I will eat." I was making a joke.

He knew I couldn't eat anything, and everything in my mouth tasted the same—like burnt ashes. But he drove four hours that day, back and forth, to bring me the fajitas I like.

I couldn't hold my tears. "You know, my love, I can't eat a thing."

He answered, "Even if the smell of it makes you smile, that's enough for me."

I was so happy at this moment. Nothing had changed his love for me; he loved me even more.

Finally, I finished the five days. Remon asked our friends to pick me up from the hospital because he was at work. I was so happy, and I longed to go home. While my friends were waiting to take me home and were talking to me, my neck started hurting and twitching. We heard this sound as if something broke. Then my head fell between my legs. It felt like someone had a very sharp knife and had started to brutally strike and twist all my bones. I screamed loudly; the nurses came running. No one understood what was happening; I couldn't speak from the pain. I just screamed.

They decided to take me down for scans. To move me while I was having this horrific pain, it was beyond any words I can describe. My face was down; I saw Neveen's legs literally shake and hit each other loudly, as if she was watching a horror movie. I told her to leave, and I refused to let her come down with me for the scans.

At this moment, I prayed for God to have mercy on me. I specifically asked Him to take my soul to let me die. I told Him, *I don't blame You for this pain, but I cannot stand it anymore; just let this end, please, God, I beg You.*

I heard Him reply in the midst of my desperation and hopelessness. He reminded me of a prayer I said many years ago. In that prayer, I told Him I didn't want a normal life. I wanted Him to shape me in His way. I wanted to have the life He planned for me. *I want my life to serve the purpose you have prepared for me.* That day, at the age of 19, I prayed these words for hours, saying the same thing over and over again.

At this point, I realized that this was not the end of my life; there would be more to come. I stopped asking God to take my life. Instead, I asked Him to give me the ability to endure the pain and to enlighten the doctors to determine the problem and resolve it.

God didn't disappoint me; they found that it was a reaction from the Compazine—nausea medicine—that made my muscles twitch, plus a blood clot had formed from the port. It took around six hours to resolve this clot.

The doctors said that everything was fine now, and they would do their best for that not to happen again. However, it happened to me two more times that night; the same exact thing happened, but these times it took less time for them to resolve it. We had to stay two more days. I felt so drained; I desperately wanted to go home.

We finally left the hospital after seven days. I was so fatigued and couldn't move at all, but I was happy to just go home.

CHAPTER 28

I Know that was YOU
Neveen

November 2017

She started to scream, "My neck! My neck hurts!"

Suddenly, Dalia's neck started to bend. All her muscles twitched. Her body shook. She screamed louder. Doctors ran here and there, fixing machines into her body, giving her tons of more medications.

Remon was not there; he had to work that day. That was to be the last day of chemotherapy for Dalia. Her friends, Hani and Lillian, had come to take her home.

"Get her out of the room!" Dalia screamed at the doctor. "Get Neveen out of the room," she yelled again.

I didn't understand. "What's wrong, dear? Let me stay with you," I said.

"No! Can't you feel? Your legs are shaking! Your legs are literally shaking. Something is going to happen to you," she screamed.

I ran to the bathroom; I needed to collapse! I needed to cry; I was scared. I felt abandoned, and

I needed to be weak, to pour out my tired soul, and to be vulnerable. Then I saw Lillian, Dalia's friend. She was in the bathroom crying too. Our eyes met. She pulled me into her arms and hugged me. I cried. I cried like I have never cried before. If I had any strength left in me, those six hours took it all away.

"Dalia will not be going home today," her doctor said, so Hani and Lillian left.

I was panicking, yet I had to be there. I had to talk with the doctors in a foreign language that I didn't know very well. And Dalia was almost having a seizure and couldn't talk for herself.

"Where do you come from, Ms. Neveen?" the doctor asked.

"From Cairo, Egypt."

"Oh, my God! Really?" he said in a Jordanian accent.

It was so good to be able to communicate with someone in my own language.

And that was when I thanked God so much. This doctor was sent from the heavens. It was not a coincidence. He could speak my language, and he could understand me. For the first time in hours, I felt hopeful. I felt I was not alone, that doctor was there to comfort me and tell me it was going to be okay, and finally, it was okay.

Then Dalia's neck started to hurt again. But

when the third round of twitches hit my sister, the Jordanian doctor was there, so this time, I was less worried.

I had to fake being all right all the time. I couldn't let Remon or Dalia see me weak; I couldn't let them see me cry! I had to be strong; I had to smile to their faces, and I had to be supportive. *How can I complain? Do I even have the right to complain? It is hard enough for everyone, and I don't want to make it harder! Not for Dalia, who's being literally crushed on all levels; not on Remon, who's witnessing the love of his life fade away, not on Rafik, my husband, my everything, who's completely helpless because I'm far away. Not on my kids, who are already suffering enough; they are too young to be left all alone. And certainly, not on my mom who's very ill and who needs me, and not on my family who are worried sick about my sister.*

I was overwhelmed. A thousand miles away from home, far, far away from my familiar comfort zone, far away from my husband, my Youssef and my Mony, apart from my family and my friends. I had no one to talk to, no one to soothe me, no one to turn to when I was about to break down. I was not surrounded by love.

I was completely devastated; it almost felt like I lost parts of me. Something died inside of me, and I couldn't bring it back to life. Agony overtook me; I wasn't just "sad." Sad was a happy adjective in my case. It was beyond that; I was drowning in my

sorrow, my helplessness, and my heartache. Do you know how it feels to wait for the next disaster? That was it; I was always scared, always expecting pain! I was tired, and I was disappointed.

My spoiled little sister, the most fashionable of us all, who took care of herself, of her beauty, of her skin, her hair, and her style, looked like a ghost in front of me. She was pale! Her skin looked weird, and it hit me so hard to see her hands. Her skin was dry and scaly; like the skin of an 80-year-old woman. *These are not my sister's hands. How could this happen to her? What kind of cure would ruin the body like that? What is it curing exactly? It is only destroying my sister.* Thoughts ran through my head; it was hard to grasp this. It was hard to understand why my sister had to look so feeble, pale, and almost lifeless.

However, while I was being tortured, while I was pretending to be fine, while I was losing pieces of my soul, this verse came to me: "Likewise the Spirit helps us in our weakness. For we do not know what to pray for as we ought, but the Spirit himself intercedes for us with groanings too deep for words" (*Romans 8:26*).

I never lost hope. I believed that the Dalia

we knew and loved would come back to us; I believed she would live, and it was Him who made me so sure of this. Because even when I couldn't speak, when I couldn't sleep or eat, and even when I tried to unite with her in her pain, I never lost hope. Even in those moments when death seemed so near.

Why, God? Why would you let this happen to her? I couldn't think right; I didn't know what to do.

And when people decided to be there for me, they were *miserable comforters.*

The phone calls never stopped; people did not understand we needed to get some sleep. They were all worried, and it put me under a lot of pressure. In our Egyptian culture, it's rude not to answer these calls; you have to. It's part of their duty to call, and you must accept it, and, in fact, return the same favor to them when they need this.

Remon did the total opposite. He didn't pick up; he ignored the calls. He stated this clearly, "I'm not going to answer. It's a tough time, and people need to understand."

But I couldn't do that. And they were, indeed, miserable comforters.

Once I was told, "I know someone who did chemotherapy before, and she went straight back to her home. Why are you making it such a big deal? Why are you staying this long at the hospital each time?" They also said tougher things like, "Neveen went to the U.S. because Dalia is dying, so she needs to bring the body back to Egypt to be buried in her family's homeland." Every time, despite everything and anything that was said, I thanked the callers for their call and hung up.

However, there were some phone calls that gave me hope. Joseph, a friend of the family, called once to pray with us on the phone. On that day, he prayed for Dalia's skin. We hadn't told him that her skin was falling off; we hadn't told anyone, so hearing him pray for this very particular thing, encouraged me. On Tuesdays, Eman and Sarah, our friends in Egypt, held weekly prayer meetings for Dalia. It meant so much to us.

God never failed to draw a smile on our faces because even during the darkest of times, He did those very little things that kept us going.

One of these "little" things came in the form of a stranger. She had a calling to visit the sick. She came into our room with a huge teddy bear. I will never forget how Dalia's face lit up on seeing this. She was so happy.

I was happy too and grateful. I looked at *this friend who's closer than a brother*, then I looked out the hospital window at the sky, and smiled. "Thank You. I know that was You." I whispered.

CHAPTER 29

Rock Bottom
Remon

November 21, 2017

When we went back to the hospital for the second chemo, this time was different. Dalia had shaved her head.

The first time she was there, she had very long hair. She looked different, however, this time she looked like cancer had broken her.

She started to belong more and more to the patients there. My brain still refused to believe that cancer could kill my wife. And yet, it seemed like cancer was winning.

We were walking this road because it was our *only* option, not because it was the best route. It was either this or give up and wait for her to die slowly.

The whole chemo session started again; a full week of treatment while being tied to her bed with all those infusions. This time, I couldn't take off another week from work.

I had to leave on Saturday at dawn; she was to be discharged Sunday. I asked my friends to pick her up and I would meet her at home on Sunday.

On my way out from work on Saturday, I called Neveen who said Dalia hadn't eaten anything since I had left. I spoke to Dalia. She said she couldn't eat any hospital food, and she couldn't wait to get home to eat from her favorite neighborhood restaurant. I decided to grab her dinner from this restaurant and took it to the hospital. She could only eat a couple bites, but I was so happy to do something that made her eat. That night, she finally ate something. I had to work the next morning and I had to drive 200 miles after a long shift, but I was so happy; she was too.

On Sunday, while at work, I got a phone call from the nurse that Dalia had an allergic reaction. They did some scans to see what was wrong with her neck. They found three clots. "Chemotherapy makes blood thicker and increases the chances for blood clots," she said.

They gave her steroids for the allergic reaction and started treating the clots right away. She was better then, but they would keep her another night and added blood thinners to her maintenance drugs.

I couldn't process the information; it was a quick phone call but full of news that I didn't expect. I don't know how I finished my shift that day. I almost wasn't seeing anything.

I called her nurse once I got off work. The

doctor said they believed the allergy was caused by Compazine, a nausea medication. They had stopped this medicine and were injecting her with steroids and Benadryl.

I spoke to Neveen. "We are all tired," she said. "You should go home, rest, and come pick us up tomorrow morning. You have to be awake and well rested to drive."

I went home, had some sleep, and early the next morning I drove to the hospital to pick her up. What I didn't know was that she had two more allergy events during the night. I couldn't stop blaming myself for not being there.

"Call to me and I will answer you."
Jeremiah 33:3

CHAPTER 30

A Change in Numbers
Dalia

November 2017

I was so careful when I got home this time. I took all the medications and the injections around the clock and tried to keep my immunity from going down.

But it seemed like there was no escape. In fact, I didn't have the luxury to spend even one day at home. I developed a fever and my white blood cell count was almost zero. The pain was horrible; I had to rush to the emergency room near my home fast. I couldn't hold my tears; it looked like I was surrounded by misery and death.

I knew my sister had to return to Egypt before Christmas. *What would I do without her?* She not only helped me with everything, but also lifted me up and kept me going. *Who could fill the void she will leave? Who could spend these days with me in the third chemo session?* She witnessed me through each change, but her love for me never changed.

I spent three more days in this hospital. On the third day, I was alone. Remon was at work, and

Neveen had to go home to get something for me. I asked to meet with the doctor.

"Can you please discharge me?" I asked.

"No," she said. "I am very sorry. You can't leave today. We did a complete blood count (CBC), and your white blood count is one. It should be at least four before you leave."

God, help me, I told Him. *I really need to go home. I have had enough pain; I need to stay away from the hospital for a few days before my next chemo cycle.* Then I asked the doctor to repeat the test.

She replied, "Why? There is no reason to do that!"

I cried, begging her to do it one more time. I told her, "I believe you will find something different. I am really tired, and I need to spend some time at home before I go back to Moffitt next week."

She finally agreed. During the time of taking another sample and waiting for them to analyze it, I prayed for a change in the count. I believed that He would do this for me. *He will give me the break I need.*

And to the doctor's surprise, she came back to me with the new numbers. "This is so strange. Your number was one; now it's six. I never expected that! Now I can let you go home."

God is here; God is near, and God listens to my tears.

When I got home, I continued reading the book of Job. It helped me during my journey of pain. He described the pain he was going through. "What is my strength, that I should wait? And what is my end, that I should be patient? Is my strength the strength of stones, or is my flesh bronze? Have I any help in me, when resource is driven from me?" (**Job 6:11-13**)

I was amazed reading this because these were my exact feelings. How amazing that was to have someone describe my exact pain without embellishments! To have someone speak for me; to have someone feel my pain. It gave me great comfort. It wiped the tears of my soul. I thanked the Lord for the book of Job and for sending me home. Then, finally, I slept—for a couple hours.

"How long will you torment me and break me in pieces with words?"
Job 19:2

CHAPTER 31

Hodor
Dalia

December 2017

Incurable disease, loneliness, depression, and death.

Dear caregiver, do not wait for any hope or optimism about tomorrow from a patient under pain, whose suffering does not end. The minutes pass like days and days like years. Death for him/her is a wish, and life is like hell. Be compassionate and do not give them more than they can endure. They don't have the ability to bear any more than their pain; they are totally powerless and vulnerable.

I told God *my body is literally falling apart. My pain is unbearable. I have no power left in me to continue this horrible type of chemo. Please, find me another way. I cannot take it anymore.*

Neveen was preparing to return to Egypt before Christmas. Her flight date was during my third chemo session, which meant I would be all alone. *How can I do this? I can't even stand by myself. I know You are here, God. I know you listen to my prayers. I believe You will find another way for me.*

I know I have the faith of a child, so when we were preparing ourselves for the third chemo, I didn't pack anything—no clothes—nothing. I trusted Him! I believed His promise: "God is faithful, and He will not let you be tempted beyond your ability."

Neveen and Remon packed their bags. Then we left for the hospital.

My oncologist ordered a CT scan before I started this chemo session. We waited in the doctor's office for the results. Remon was so worried and a little excited to hear if this chemo had done anything good. While for me, all I thought about, at this moment, was that I could not continue this medication.

When my oncologist came into the room, he said, "Dalia, I have some news for you. One of them is bad, and the other one might be good."

I asked, "What is the bad news?"

"The chemo you have been taking is not working," he said. "Your tumor has grown."

When he said that, Remon was shocked, but I smiled.

My doctor was confused. "Do you understand what I just said?"

"Yes," I said. *This means I won't continue*

this treatment. God heard my prayers.

Then he told us about the good news. "It's a new immunotherapy treatment. We found a gene mutation in your tumor that may work with this type of treatment. We still don't know much about this medicine. Few people have tried it; you will be one of them. But we need approval from your insurance. This treatment is very expensive, and the results are not that great yet."

The doctor explained the plan. "You will take this treatment, plus one type of chemotherapy. You can leave the hospital the same day you have the treatment."

That was amazing. I knew it would be a lot of driving, but for me, I was so happy to change the treatment.

We returned home the same day. Remon was unpacking our bag, and he asked me, "Where are your clothes?"

I answered. "I didn't pack anything."

He asked, "Why?"

I told him. "I asked God not to give me anything beyond what I was able to endure because I couldn't take it anymore."

Neveen flew back to Egypt.

I was so fatigued and weak. Remon continued to read a lot about this new treatment and talked to the insurance company.

People started to text me, telling me awful things.

"Why are you resisting God's will for you?"

"Your tumor got bigger. Why do you insist on continuing with treatment?"

"If He had wanted to heal you, He would have done it in a second."

"It is so obvious He doesn't want to heal you, so why do you keep on torturing yourself with lousy medications?"

"Stop resisting God's will and don't be stubborn."

However, I believe that God works in everything; *He can heal anything; He can create a medicine just for me.* I didn't listen to these people's words.

Until I got this call—this weird call. Someone's way of showing empathy was to make me worry about Remon and how he should continue his life after I die. I was shocked; I couldn't speak. Inside me, I was furious. I couldn't breathe. The phone dropped from my hand. *How could you say that? How dare you? Now you made me think about the darkest scenarios. You threw my mind into a dreadful place. I wasn't thinking about that at all. Why did you do that to me? Remon is the love of my life. Why must you crush my soul like this?*

I started to have nightmares. I felt death was surrounding me. I started to lose hope. I even told my oncologist, "I am thinking about death all the time."

He referred me to a psychiatrist. She was awesome, and she gave me antidepressants. She said, "Just speak to the people who really care about you. Refuse all the negative thoughts to keep going."

Soon after that, I was home alone, screaming out in pain. I tried to go to the restroom by myself. Remon was at work, and Mays was not there. Finally, I made it to the bathroom; the pain was horrible. Then I started to bleed. I cried loudly. I needed help, but I was alone.

Hodor, my dog, heard me. He came running and found me crying; he tried to cheer me up, but the pain was unbearable. He went to the living room, started grabbing all his toys, and brought them to the restroom to make me stop crying. Then with his cute face holding one of his toys, he pushed it toward me. Then he hugged me. That felt amazing. As if he was saying to me *you are not alone.*

CHAPTER 32
A Non-Covered Test
Remon

December 2017

I checked my mailbox that day and grabbed a bunch of letters. Sitting at my desk, I started going through them. They were mostly hospital bills. I filed them in my bills file.

It was so easy to miss a payment, so I started a tight filing system: paid, pending, or to be disputed. "Paid" meant I made the payment and was covered by insurance. "Pending" meant the final decision was made and it was either covered or rejected, but it still needed to be paid, and probably we didn't have the money for it right now. "Dispute" meant it was not covered, either because insurance didn't cover the services or because it needed adjustment from the hospital or justification from the doctor like when she stayed for seven days for chemo and the initial authorization was only for five days.

These piles became overwhelming. Like we didn't have enough already with everything we were going through. Keeping up with the bills meant making a lot of phone calls to the insurance and billing department of the hospital regarding each statement. I was exhausted. I had to juggle work, taking care of my sick wife, keeping track of payments, and not falling in debt. I looked at my pending payments stack and realized it was getting bigger.

It was Christmas time, and everyone was buying Christmas presents, one more thing I needed to budget for. I suddenly realized that we were going to miss Christmas that year. Dalia was receiving her treatment; we would not be able to leave home or go anywhere to celebrate Christmas. I was afraid that this might be the last Christmas for us together.

It was at this time that I found a bill that stopped my train of thoughts; it was almost $7,000, and it was not covered by insurance. That was the insurance's final decision; we had to pay it. That statement was for a genomic profiling test to analyze Dalia's DNA and look for genetic mutations. I tried to remember when we had this test done. I vaguely remembered that this test was ordered in April 2017 by Dalia's previous oncologist before the very first recurrence.

I didn't have the breath nor the clear mind that day to start making phone calls to fight this bill. But I did make one phone call to Dalia's current oncologist office. I asked his nurse to transfer these results to their office and have Dr. R review it.

She said, "The doctor will discuss the test results on your next visit, but for the meantime, nothing should change. The protocol Dalia's following is the first line of treatment in her case."

It was time for the third chemo session and another scan needed to be done. After two rounds of chemo, Dalia's oncologist wanted to see if the treatment had made any progress. For the last six weeks, I saw Dalia start to fade. Chemo was like a monster chewing her up slowly. But I always told myself *If the treatment was that bad, it should be doing something.*

On our way to the hospital, Dalia was literally dragging. She didn't want to go this time; this chemo was worse than cancer she said.

I tried to look for some light, even a tiny bit of good news. I hoped that the tumor had shrunk. But Dalia only thought about stopping the treatment.

The doctor announced the results. "Dalia, your tumor got bigger even with our *best chemo*."

I was shocked; everything I had hoped for just collapsed. If their *best chemo* was not working, I guessed nothing would work.

The doctor continued. "These results are not far from what we expected though; the chances were so little after all."

I looked at Dalia for any reaction, but she was quiet. She seemed even relieved that she didn't have to continue this treatment. She wanted to stop at any cost, even if this meant the treatment would fail and the tumor would grow.

Then the doctor said, "This actually might not be the end; I reviewed the DNA test results that you called about." He continued. "We actually have a new option now. The genomic profiling test showed some genetic mutations in Dalia's tumor which may respond to one new immunotherapy medication called Olaratumab. After reviewing your test results, Olaratumab might be an option. The side effects won't be as bad as the current treatment, and Dalia won't have to stay at the hospital for five days every time."

I asked him, "Is it *an* option or *a good* option?" I remembered that ifosfamide was our *only* option before, and the results were not good at all. We couldn't keep pushing her into different treatments without any good outcome in sight.

He answered, "The new medication is being tested for sarcoma patients specifically with Dalia's gene mutation. Some studies show increased life expectancy with Olaratumab. There are no solid final results yet, but there are many studies taking place in different hospitals that will provide more information soon, and Dalia will be in one of those studies."

I looked at Dalia; we didn't say anything.

The doctor noticed our confusion, so he tried to explain, "The new treatment protocol will be a combo of Olaratumab infusion followed by doxorubicin. The cycle will be two weeks of Olaratumab in a row, one week with doxorubicin and one week without. Then one-week break without meds before the new cycle begins." Then, in an encouraging tone, he said to Dalia, "You don't have to stay in the hospital for the treatment. You can go home the same day. Just use Neulasta to inject yourself at home; this will help your white blood cell count to go up after each doxorubicin session."

We didn't know what to say. We were tired of all this information. Dalia asked for some time to think.

That time I couldn't push Dalia toward the treatment as I had before. She had those surgeries and painful chemo because I refused to let her give up, and yet we ended up here. On the inside, my hopes evaporated. In the past, my hopes were high before every scan or any treatment option we had discussed. But after two surgeries and horrible chemotherapy, nothing had happened. It was always the worst-case scenario.

We were unable to decide. We had received really bad news—again—and at the same time a new door opened. Could it bring better results this time? Or would we be wasting our last days together in the hospital. I freaked out thinking this really might be our last Christmas.

*"Pray for one another, that you may be healed.
The prayer of a righteous person has great
power as it is working."*
James 5:16

CHAPTER 33

The Weak—The Strong
Dalia

December 2017

I was so confused during this time. *What is that new medicine?* I had a lot of questions and got zero answers. They didn't know its side effects yet, or even if it would work. Not enough patients had used it, so there was very little information about it. The Food and Drug Administration (FDA) had expedited the approval process because there were no other medications for sarcoma on the market yet.

However, John, my wonderful friend from North Carolina, started an online prayer group for me. Prayers were offered from so many different parts of the world. They fasted and prayed for me. I shared the news with them and asked the group to pray for my next step.

After a few days, one of the members of the group sent me a voice message. "Dalia, I prayed for you a lot, and I wanted to tell you that God's voice was so clear. The Lord will do twice as many times as that medicine could possibly do. God has a powerful story for you. It's not the end. Keep having faith in that and keep going."

That was amazing! He gave me great hope. I remembered back when they told me if the tumor didn't respond to this chemo then it would be the end for me. But, at least now, they were giving me another hope. I could see how God had blessed me with my oncologist, Dr. R. He and his team worked, researched, and studied for me. They encouraged me to not give up.

Then I found a lot of other messages sent from people I barely knew, and some others, whom I didn't know at all. They told me about a prayer meeting that took place at my church in Egypt, led by my spiritual leader Dr. Sameh. They had been touched by my story. They prayed, and many surrendered their lives to God. And then they prayed for healing for me. These messages were so touching; I couldn't hold back my tears reading them.

Then my best friend Deena from Egypt told me about this meeting and how powerful it was. And how everyone cried and prayed from their hearts. Not just this, she told me that there were two other churches praying for me at the same time from different cities in Egypt. To know *I am not alone; I have a prayer army who has my back, believing in God's hand, begging, and asking for a miracle for ME* was a great joy and a source of hope for my next step.

I prepared myself for the new treatment. I knew this time, most of the days I would be home alone. Remon's shifts were very long. I started to think about the patients who had to be in this fight with no one around them at all; no one to pray for them, and sometimes it looks like they have no reason to go on. I found that these people are much braver and stronger; they fight this battle alone.

Dr. Sameh, the one who led that prayer meeting in Egypt wrote these words:

"When our church decided to hold a prayer meeting for Dalia, I was asked to lead the meeting. Despite the fact that I never led a prayer meeting before, I agreed, because I was so close to Dalia and Remon. I had a certain message from God that I wanted to deliver—about Dalia's healing. A huge number of people came. It was unexpected because that was unusual compared to the normal prayer meetings. It felt like God really wanted to do something on that night. My major focus was on how God performs miracles on a daily basis. I mentioned that God wanted us to ask Him for a miracle. People listened carefully; they were enthusiastic, and they were eager for the time of prayer. I read these words for the prayer group; 'So Peter rose and went with them. And when he arrived, they took him to the upper room. All the widows stood beside him weeping and showing tunics and other garments that Dorcas made while she was with them' (**Acts 9:39**)."

Dr. Sameh continued. "As I read these words, I couldn't stop myself. Tears fell down my face; I couldn't speak for a few minutes. I looked at all the faces; they were Dalia's friends. They loved her; served God with her. Then I uttered these words: those women in the scripture showed Peter the clothes Dorcas made for them, and we can do the same now. We can share with God and with each other what Dalia did among us, and we can declare that God is able to heal her, and He will. We took some time, and we prayed in groups, and everyone prayed, cried, and believed in the miracle to come."

- Sameh Samy, Egypt.

Knowing all of this got me thinking about that question: This is a battle; so which team will you choose?

In this battle, two teams will surround you. One team has negative thoughts and words that desire to put you down or even crush your soul. The other team lifts you up, supports you, prays for you, and gives you hope and positive energy. That team will help you keep going to win your battle.

I decided to shut the door to all those who

wanted to discourage me, even if some of their words sounded true. I decided to listen to the people who really loved me; who prayed with faith for support and healing.

Dear reader, open your heart to see beyond what others can see, to see beyond your disease, your problems, your difficult situation. God is working and He is bigger than your pain. He is bigger than your grief. Look up to the sky and let Him be in your life. You will realize who is in control. You will realize that you are not surrounded by cancer. You are not surrounded by your problems, sadness, or loneliness. *He* surrounds your whole life despite any complication you may have. At some point, many people believed that cancer was defeating me— that there was no way out. But in my darkest moments, I came to Him and I saw a whole different scenario.

If you are fighting this battle alone, I encourage you to find a support group. Search for someone who can give you the support you need. Think about something you love to do; something you want to accomplish. Search for a new hope, a new will to live, a reason to keep going, to keep fighting. You are here for a reason; you are not just a number in this life. You are unique; you are God's son, God's daughter. And if there is no one else around, *He* is here and *He* is in control.

Life is not easy. Every one of us has his/her own battle to fight. And you are the only one who's able to choose victory or to choose defeat. You are the one who is capable of choosing the weak or the strong position to fend off the attacks of this illness.

In our battle, the people normally perceived as strong in their daily life are not always powerful in this fight against cancer, and those who are considered weak aren't always the ones who give up the fight. Because in this battle, the weak is the one who gives up without fighting back, and the strong is the one who totally trusts and leans on God's promises.

"You are altogether beautiful, my love;
there is no flaw in you."
Song of Solomon 4:7

CHAPTER 34
An Inside Out Change
Dalia

January 2018

Flowery cute dresses, ruffle tops, girly skirts! That's all I could find when I looked in my closet. Even my accessories are very sophisticated. I sat on the floor and cried for hours. *Why? Nothing will look good on me. I am so different than I was before chemo. I can't wear any of my clothes now.* But a thought hit me. *Change!* I heard it clearly in my mind. *Maybe I need to change my style. I can enjoy every moment of my life. I can turn a disaster into something beautiful.*

I called Mays, and we went shopping. We had a great time. I created a very nice new style. I was so happy. I even took some selfies and shared them with my siblings and friends.

On that day, I started to see my situation from a totally different angle. I saw myself and God in a different way: so clear, so pure. Through Him, I realized a new aspect of beauty. For the first time in my life, I recognized how pretty and confident I was. I didn't need beautiful hair. I didn't need perfect skin to be able to step outside my door to face the world. I could see my beauty through my scars and through the quiet smile on my face despite the pain and the bad news. Because I could feel His presence.

I am surrounded by His strength and peace. I finally realize that my value is in Him. I am the daughter of the King of Kings. Now I can look in the mirror and see a pretty fighter who knows very well her worth and who she really is. I am that perfectly cut, unique diamond. Neither cancer nor the devil himself can break me. I don't care if I will live or die because I know my place and my value. Cancer cannot change that. I will accept and love myself. I'm not going to hide. I'm not going to feel ashamed to meet anyone with the way I look now. And this was when I decided to never wear my wig again.

I won't lie to you. It was very surprising to me. Because only a few days before, the situation was totally different. I was a mess. I thought of how everyone was celebrating their Christmas. Decorations and Christmas trees were everywhere; people were on holidays, meeting up in family gatherings and sharing gifts with their loved ones. While on the other hand, there I was, in the hospital starting my new treatment— starting another path to walk through with a different type of pain, going back and forth every week to Moffitt, to keep fighting my battle.

As I walked to my new hospital room to get ready for my session, my eyes fell on *that* thing: the bell. What was that doing here? Could something so small help ease my huge pain? Could it make a difference for someone like me? Nothing, literally nothing, worked for me. *What are my chances to ever ring that bell?*

One day, after the new treatment started, I felt dizzy. I felt so much fatigue, nausea, and heartburn. *Only God knows how my body is shaking, how my bones ache as if somebody is grinding them.* Home alone, trying so hard to get up from my bed. I couldn't. I waited for an hour, hoping to feel better. I was thirsty; my lips were so dry they hurt.

I tried to encourage myself. *Come on, Dalia, you can do it.* I put my hands on my bed and tried to push my body forward, but it didn't work. I started to count the steps from my bed to the kitchen. I cried out to God. I felt there were countless steps to make. After a couple of hours, I could finally get up. I walked, filled a cup, and, oh, it felt so good.

Then I opened my eyes—to find it was only a dream. I was still in my bed, in desperate need of a cup of water. After many failed attempts, I decided to wait until Remon came home from work. That day I waited 12 hours to quench my thirst.

Desperation overtook me. I couldn't hold my tears, remembering how active I used to be. Now, a girl in her 20s, living her days like a very old, helpless woman. Not just physically; this girl had also lost all beauty she used to have. She can't even recognize herself when she looks in the mirror.

But in the middle of this sadness, I started to think about the very simple things I used to do every day; things I used to take for granted. Now doing these things felt like a very big deal. I found myself praying, talking about how thankful I am, for I can breathe. I was thankful that my tumor hadn't reached my lungs yet, thankful for keeping my faith in the middle of this madness and thankful for every day I had the chance to walk, run, travel, and laugh without feeling pain. I decided then, and I promised God, that anytime I could move, I would enjoy it. I promised to do something different; something that I liked.

The girl who looked desperately at that bell was the same girl who could change her style. The girl who had a dream she was drinking a cup of water was the same girl who thanked God in the midst of pain, and it was all because of Him. He was preparing me for the next step: new scans. It was time to know if my new treatment was making any difference at all.

"But who are you, O man, to answer back to God? Will what is molded say to its molder, 'Why have you made me like this?'"
Romans 9:20

CHAPTER 35

The "Why"
Dalia

I was very surprised with the number of people who had "why" questions. Some of them were struggling with death; however, some of them were simply young people, just starting their lives. They both asked me: WHY?

Why withstand all that pain?

Why fight death?

Why decide to take chemo, when it had a very low chance of success?

Why? **Is life worth all that?**

I fully understood the thoughts of young people encountering pain, face to face. They were justified questions after all. But what I didn't understand was the perception and comments of others who didn't experience suffering.

And it was my turn to ask:

Why be hopeless?

Why give up so quickly?

I'm not saying life is totally worth it; I'm not saying it is a piece of cake. But our lives are worth living to the maximum, even if only for a few more months, or weeks, or hours.

Don't put a full stop to your story. The world is cruel; it's full of pain and evil. Giving up is the easiest option.

But God is able to make a change. He is capable of changing evil to good.

Guess what? Cancer was not the worst thing that happened to me. But I had this habit of running to His arms whenever I faced a trauma.

It was a rough journey—sometimes.

I lost hope!

I screamed!

I cried like never before!

But I never ever doubted His goodness!

"Let no one say when he is tempted, 'I am being tempted by God' for God cannot be tempted with evil, and he himself tempts no one." *(James 1:13)*

He can fix all that is broken, and for that, I will allow Him to add more lines to my story. When a full stop is to put an end to my story, in His timing, I will be the happiest, for I will know I never gave up.

CHAPTER 36
The Gray Area
Remon

February 2018

The new treatment combo was definitely more tolerable than the ifosfamide. It still had side effects, and it wasn't easy at all, but it wasn't eating her alive.

After two cycles, it was time for another scan. I lost count of how many scans Dalia had to do since all this began. I started to wonder if all these scans could be harmful. Then I realized how silly the question was with all the side effects she was already experiencing with every round of chemotherapy.

My hopes grew with every scan only to fall into frustration. Because the immunotherapy's side effects were reasonable this time, I had a feeling that it might not be working at all. I tried not to be overly anxious. But as usual, I couldn't sleep at night either. I couldn't sleep the night before any scan for a full year.

The moment finally came. For the first time ever, we had good news. The tumor had shrunk, and finally, it had responded to the immunotherapy. For the first time in months, I felt like I could breathe again.

"Now is the best time to have a surgery to remove this tumor," the oncologist said. "Four months ago, it was inoperable, and it didn't make sense to keep operating on a tumor that kept coming back."

When we first met Dalia's doctor, he refused the idea of a surgery at all, but now he said we might have a chance while the tumor was localized and condensed. He asked if we had any questions.

"Will removing the tumor be the cure?" I asked.

"The tumor came back several times; we don't know if it will continue to do so." The doctor paused. "But for the first time, we have a treatment that is working, and we have a chance to be ahead of the tumor after being behind in the past. We will continue our treatment protocol four weeks after surgery." The doctor was so happy with the results; we felt that we personally meant a great deal to him.

Dalia and I were excited. For the first time, we could smile after a scan; we finally felt there may be some light at the end.

The oncologist's team set us up with a surgeon. He was so thorough explaining everything to Dalia. So thorough that Dalia started to freak out again. She became reluctant about having the surgery, after knowing how extreme it would be. The surgeon planned to remove anything adjacent to or that had been touched by the tumor. This included not only the tumor itself, but also her kidney, her diaphragm, and part of her stomach.

She was not ready for a huge surgery of this kind again; she had already experienced so much pain. This would be her third surgery at the same spot.

"The healing process this time will be even slower," the doctor said. "Your multiple chemotherapy treatments will slow down the healing."

We experienced all kinds of mixed emotions. We didn't know if we should be happy because the treatment was finally working or to be worried because the tumor may come back. We didn't know if we should be excited because the surgery was a promising option or angry because this was the third time she had to go through this kind of pain. Trying to process all these feelings overwhelmed us; nothing seemed to come without strings attached.

There was not one absolutely good option that would solve our problems. Our options were always in the gray area. Every time, we had to discover the new extent of pain she could endure and wait for results that might or might not be good.

"Thus, the Lord used to speak to Moses face to face, as a man speaks to his friend."
Exodus 33:11

". . . let me see your face, let me hear your voice, for your voice is sweet, and your face is lovely."
Song of Solomon 2:14

CHAPTER 37
An Agreement
Dalia

Memorizing all the verses, implementing the commandments, praying all the time, listening to His Word, and doing what's right; isn't it enough?!

What God wants from you and me is much simpler, but also, much more complicated than this.

When I read the story of Jesus cleansing ten lepers in *Luke 17:11-19*, I wondered why Jesus felt bad. Yes, only one came back and thanked Jesus, but the rest of the lepers did exactly what Jesus asked them to do. They did not only listen to Him, but they also believed His words and all of them went to the priest and followed His instructions without questioning. Jesus didn't ask them to thank Him. But He wanted them to do that because what Jesus wants is a relationship.

"Thank you." How simple those words were, but those words showed more significance, a deeper meaning in how He wanted more than just following the instructions.

February 2018

I waited in my oncologist's office. Too many thoughts raced through my head. I really wanted good news—any good news—but what if this treatment was not working. That would be our last chance in this battle. My hands were freezing and I could hardly breathe.

Dr. R entered the room with the results in his hand and a nice smile on his face. "Dalia, finally, I have good news for you. The new treatment has worked and your tumor has shrunk."

I couldn't believe what I just heard. We finally heard something good. *There is hope.* It was an amazing moment.

But Dr. R continued. He spoke about another surgery. "While this treatment did shrink the tumor, it is still very aggressive and we shouldn't underestimate it. Now we have a chance to remove it and continue the treatment afterwards."

Another surgery; another incision, another pain, and the long healing process. I thought the new medicine had worked, and now I would experience less pain. But the doctors saw it as an opportunity to remove the tumor while it was smaller. I started to accept the idea of the surgery because of the new treatment outcome—until we met the surgeon.

"This surgery will not be easy at all," he said. "I will have to remove your left kidney, your diaphragm, part of your stomach and anything else that the tumor touched. And there is no guarantee that it will not come back. There is also no guarantee that I will be able to clean everything out." He paused. "There are possible complications. If your body rejects the new tissue which replaces the diaphragm, and if a leak occurs in your stomach, you might have to live with a tube in your nose, by which you would eat and drink for the rest of your life."

He mentioned too many other things, and I started to feel so concerned about the idea of this surgery. Especially with what I had already experienced before. The decision was so hard to make; they were waiting for my answer.

I decided to pray. I told God what was worrying me about this surgery. That I didn't want to live the rest of my life with more health complications. I talked to Him for hours. Then I started to thank Him for what the treatment did with my tumor; I thanked Him for being with me the whole journey, for having this peaceful feeling inside my heart all the time, for correcting the false and mistaken thoughts about His love for me, for shaping and forming my mind and for showing me how much faith, strength, and beauty I have within me. Then I asked Him for healing—for an end to this pain. I asked Him for mercy—for a miracle.

While I was praying, God told me to share my fears and my faith with the prayer group that my friend John started. I shared with them the updates, then I found myself telling them that I believed God would not let me undergo this surgery.

"I am praying and I know that God is here, and He is listening. He is still performing miracles," I told them. "I believe that He will do something different for me." I told the prayer group, "I thanked God for my healing to come, for not letting them do this surgery or remove any of these organs." I asked my friends to pray with me the same thing.

On the day of the surgery, I prayed these same words. On our way to the hospital, Remon asked me if I was fine. I answered, "Yes, I am good."

"How? Aren't you worried? It's a big surgery!"

"I am not going to do it," I said.

He freaked out, begging me not to say that to the doctors as they would not do the surgery if I told them that. They would think I was withdrawing my consent to undergo the procedure.

I calmed him down, telling him it was just an agreement between me and God. God promised me that I was not going to do it.

When we arrived at the hospital, I changed, and they took me to the operating room. I kept praying the same thing until they started the anesthesia.

CHAPTER 38

Excision
Remon

March 2018
Surgery day

I really like the movie *Groundhog Day* where the main character lives the same day over and over again. But I now started to understand how he felt. This third surgery at the same spot came with the same prep and the same incision pain and recovery afterwards. It was nerve-wracking.

They prepared her for surgery, and it was time to send me out to the waiting area. Dalia spoke to me many times about how God would not let her undergo the surgery. I knew she has always relied on her emotions more than her logic. They started to give her anesthesia meds. If anything about the surgery could change, it was too late then.

They took her to the operating room. The nurse called me every hour to give me updates about her status. After four hours, they took me to a small room to meet with the surgeon. That was a bit weird because they had reserved a longer time slot for this surgery. I started to wonder why they had finished earlier than expected. *Did something go wrong?* I didn't wait long before the surgeon entered the room.

"During the surgery, I examined samples of the removed tissues on the spot. These samples were meant to guide me on what to remove next. The quick results were great and showed the tumor was either dead or localized. I removed the tumor and part of her stomach, but I didn't have to remove the kidney or the diaphragm."

My brain tried to process. "What does this mean?" I asked.

"This is not the final pathology results yet," he said. "What we did during the surgery was a quick test and the results are not 100 percent reliable; we only use it as a guide. However, the tissues I tested were dead cancer cells."

I had so many questions.

He understood how worried I was. "I know how long your journey has been and how much Dalia has suffered so far," he said. "But this is good news. This is better than our wildest wishes, so enjoy the moment and go back to your wife. She needs you beside her when she wakes up." Then he added, "Dalia is in good health; she is recovering now. The surgery went well, and the final results will be in the pathology report."

I felt incredible. The doctor didn't remove anything he had planned to. Dalia had talked so much about how she would not have this surgery. I thought that she was a dreamer; I tried to keep pulling her back to reality. I was concerned that after high hopes would come the frustration, and she may fall into depression if I didn't always keep her hopes logical.

When they finally took me to see her, she was sleeping. She opened her eyes and asked me what happened?

"You had the surgery, but at the same time, you didn't have the surgery," I said.

"What does that mean?" Dalia asked me.

I told her what the doctor had said.

"I told you." She smiled. "I will not have this surgery." Then she went back to sleep.

"I had heard of you by the hearing of the ear,
but now my eye sees you..."
Job 42:5

CHAPTER 39

A Promise Keeper
Dalia

Many were praying for a miracle, but I felt I was already living the miracle. When I was in the midst of deep sorrow, but I had this calming peace, then, that was a miracle!

When I let go of what I loved most, and I felt okay with it, then that was a miracle!

When people all over the world, whom I had never met, from different churches, prayed for the same exact thing at the same exact time, then that was a miracle!

When people who I didn't know messaged me their stories, told me that I was a blessing to them, then, that was a miracle!

When doctors thought I wouldn't be able to move, when they believed I would collapse, but the total opposite occurred, then, that was a miracle!

To be alive until that moment was a miracle!

Sometimes, we just don't notice how our lives are full of miracles.

Think about this, be thankful to God, for all His miracles.

-Posted on my Facebook profile in January 2018

March 2018

"Do you hear me? Dalia, wake up . . . Wake up, please. There is something important I need to tell you," Remon said.

I could hardly open my eyes. I saw Remon; he looked so happy. He asked me again if I could hear him well. I was in so much pain and connected to many machines. There was also a tube in my nose to my stomach. Which made it more difficult to speak. I nodded to let him know that I could hear him.

"You almost didn't do the surgery," he said. "I don't know how, but the surgeon decided to analyze the samples he got from you in the surgery room, and he found that all your cancer cells were dead. He decided not to remove any organs as he originally planned."

My feelings were indescribable. My heart danced. There were not enough words to describe how happy I was. We both smiled and cried. Remon was jumping, and for the first time since I got sick, he started to call our families and friends sharing with them what God had done for us. And how He answered their prayers.

Oh, God! How good You are. You never

turned me down. I knew You would listen to my supplication. You would put an end to my pain and misery. I knew that You would raise me up; You would breathe life in me. When I talk about You, I speak with power, I never hesitate. Because I trusted You, for You always keep Your promises. Your love for me never changes.

We waited ten days for the final results that would be far more accurate. I had just left the hospital, so Dr. R, my oncologist, called me with the updates.

His voice was so happy telling me this remarkable news. "Dalia, all the cancer cells in your body were dead. That was beyond our expectations. I will give you three weeks to rest and recover from your surgery, then we will continue our immunotherapy and chemo combo." Then he emailed us the final pathology report.

I was officially in remission. My body was clean; God had miraculously saved me. I posted the final report on my Facebook and told all my family, friends, and everyone who had prayed for me. "God listened and He answered your prayers. Our God is alive, and He feels for our pain and He hears our sighing. There is power in His name. Call on Him and believe in His Word. Always trust His promises." I wrote.

I knew I was totally cured, but some people

I knew were overly excited and tried to convince me to completely stop the treatment. "You don't need any more medications now," they said. "You should show that you believe in God and refuse the treatment."

For them, that was a declaration of faith of some sort, but I thought that was silly. I believed God uses different ways and I believed he used medicine to heal me. Not listening to my doctor now wasn't a declaration of defeating cancer, it was empty bragging. I decided to continue the treatment and to listen to my oncologist. I really trusted him as I felt how much he cared about my health.

CHAPTER 40

Road Trips
Remon

May 2018

Our lives changed after the third surgery. Dalia took a break for a month to heal before she continued the treatment combo. She continued on Olaratumab and doxorubicin for another three months. The plan was to continue this treatment for another four months, but Dalia's heart started to have some issues, and it appeared that she couldn't tolerate the doxorubicin anymore.

She was supposed to receive eight cycles of doxorubicin, that was the maximum anyone could get in a lifetime. Even if a patient had a recurrence later, after using doxorubicin for eight cycles, they could never use it again. The doctors would have to change the medicine because after eight cycles it becomes really dangerous and harmful, especially for the heart.

The next scan results were great for the second time in a row. After these great results, the doctor decided to stop the doxorubicin after seven cycles instead of eight. That was a huge step forward for Dalia; she started to improve dramatically.

Dalia continued the immunotherapy alone for another full year afterward. We had to drive to the hospital two weeks in a row and then take a one-week break before we returned for another two weeks. It was our weekly road trip for 12 months. That schedule continued until May 2019.

"He also allured you out of distress into a broad place where there was no cramping, and what was set on your table was full of fatness."
Job 36:16

CHAPTER 41

Do You Hear the Ring?
Dalia

May 2019

For another year, I continued my treatment. My scan results every three months were always clear, and finally the day came; that day before I started my last immunotherapy session.

I met with Dr. R. He congratulated me. "I am so proud of you and the courage you had. I know this was a difficult journey, but I am so happy for you and with what we achieved together until this moment." Then he told me that the company manufacturing my immunotherapy drug was withdrawing the medication from the market because the results of the studies didn't show a significant benefit against the group of patients who received doxorubicin alone. "It's like this medication was made especially for you," he said.

I was overwhelmed with all this news. It was my last session; I couldn't believe this day had come. The day I had no more pain, no more needles, and no more dizziness or nausea. I watched the last infusion bag as it emptied into my body and couldn't believe that was actually happening. The nurse came and took the needles off my chest. I found the rest of the nurses waiting for me beside the bell. One of them handed me a certificate, which all of them had signed, that I bravely finished my treatment. I finally had the chance to ring the bell. I used to hear people ringing the bell as a sign of hope; someone was done with treatment, someone was healed and sending a message to everyone around, including me, "Go on! you can do it, you can finish it too!" I used to hear this bell and felt that my turn would never come. But now I could publicly announce that my journey with pain had come to an end.

I tried to ring the bell as hard as I could. Maybe someone who was receiving treatment in one of these rooms could hear the bell and be encouraged by me. The nurses gathered around me and hugged me while the cheers came from everywhere, it was such a joyful moment.

June 2019

My younger sister set her wedding to a later date after I had finished my last session. She had decided, two years before, to wait until I was cancer free and I was able to attend the wedding. At the airport in Egypt, I found all my friends and family waiting for me with beautiful flowers.

When I saw them, I couldn't hold back my tears. I thought this day might never come. I thought I would never see them again. I finally felt their warm hugs. That moment was worth everything in the world to me. We all celebrated the wedding; it was the best day ever, and my sister was gorgeous.

I am so thankful to my God, the Almighty Father, Who gave me life instead of death, joy instead of lamentations, praise instead of despair, and beauty instead of ashes. Now I am thankful for every new day I live, for every time I can eat something and actually taste it, for every step I can take without help, and for every day I spend at home. I am thankful for my hair, skin, and nails; for all the things I used to take for granted. Now, I really appreciate and spend hours thanking the Lord.

I finally realized that I didn't need huge things to be happy. My happiness now comes in the tiniest things in life that may seem normal for anyone else. I value my pain, and I am so thankful for this journey, *for my pain is not a waste.*

CHAPTER 42
The Phoenix
Remon

May 2019

Many things have changed in our lives.

Dalia had good scans every three months for a full year. But that was not enough to relieve my anxiety that I developed over the course of our journey. Every time we had a scan, I couldn't sleep that night at all. The doctor's advice was to learn to enjoy the moment and celebrate the good news while I could, otherwise, I would spend my life waiting for the next scan results. Honestly, I still need to learn this. I spend a lot of time worrying about things that I can't change, which makes me miss the joy that I can have in the current moment.

Also, I am still a bit isolated and not fitting with people of my age any longer. I think this experience added at least ten or more years to my life. I find myself feeling better when I'm alone. I started to not enjoy big groups of people. I learned that having one true friend, like Mays was for Dalia, is better than being surrounded by superficial relationships that don't scratch the surface of your soul.

I learned to be more compassionate with my patients. Cancer, or whatever kind of pain or health issues a person might have, is not an easy experience to go through. Everyone has a story, and I believe it is not less painful than ours.

Taking that extra step for one of my patients opened my eyes to a new treatment option for Dalia, when she told me about her husband and Moffitt Cancer Center.

I learned about God's timing. Getting an uncovered bill for the DNA test made me call the hospital and check for a different treatment option right before her current chemotherapy failed.

Dalia's getting sick at this time enabled her to receive Olaratumab; if she had become sick one year earlier or any time after April 2019, this medicine wouldn't have been available for her. The company withdrew the medication from the market because the final studies showed no significant statistical benefit for the medicine, but for Dalia it was the game changer. You can find the company's release about this medication on the Lilly Pharmaceutical website.

Now the hospital is using Dalia's case to defend patients who have a similar genetic mutation to receive the same treatment.

When everything started, I never imagined that Dalia could be this strong. She may look tiny or a bit spoiled with love sometimes, but she rose like a Phoenix from the cancer ashes. She was a warrior when she needed to be. After I almost lost her, I learned to appreciate each moment we are together.

"So they said to him,
'Then what sign do you do, that we may see and
believe you?
What work do you perform?'"
John 6:30

God Is Not Santa Claus
Dalia

Three years full of struggles, tears, loneliness, hopelessness, and pain.

"Why? He could have healed you with just one word without all this pain and damage to your body and soul."

"Why did you have to walk this path?"

"Couldn't He heal you even without this new immunotherapy?"

People ask me these questions all the time. Then I started to think about the miracles that Jesus did while He was among us on this earth. I started to rethink the process of each miracle and the steps He took and how the miracle recipients received the miracle or responded.

I remembered when He touched the leper before healing him. Yes, He could have said a word, but instead, He touched him (Mark 1:40-42). For that poor leper who had not been touched by anyone for many years, I assume that touch meant the world to him. Jesus knew what that man really needed, and how this touch would mend his soul. This man needed to feel like a human again, maybe even more than he needed the miracle itself.

This is the God whom I love. The Almighty whom I follow. He is not a show man nor a performer or a magician. He cares about me, my journey, my personality, and how I feel in every step along the way. He cares how I will grow in my relationship with Him, to get closer to Him, to be more like Him, and to reflect His image.

Before He healed my body, He had cured my soul and my wrong concepts. I experienced the miracle before it actually happened. I experienced the peace of God that surpasses all understanding while still in the peak of pain. If He gave me the healing instantly, I would have been the same person with no change. And one day, I would die missing all the blessings I received during my journey with pain. For God cares more about who I am than what I do. God cares more about who *you are* than what *you do*.

Sometimes healing is a side result, not the main purpose. I have seen a lot of people with major health problems. They never had a healing miracle nor were they totally healed. But their lives were full of miracles.

If you want your relationship with God to be all about requests and answers, you need to change your mind. Because our God is not Santa

Claus.

Did my journey have to happen in this way?

Yes, I needed that immunotherapy. It was God's plan for me. I used to live in Ohio. Then I moved to Florida one year before I had cancer. It had to be this specific medication in that specific hospital at that specific time. I was blessed to have had this type of treatment. After I had finished my sessions, the company stopped producing this medicine. The studies claimed that there were no remarkable results. I was the only case that had these great results. As if this treatment was made specifically for me, literally. My oncologist told me if I was diagnosed one year earlier or three months later, I would not have had the chance to receive that treatment.

I saw a lot of people who refused to get any treatment saying, "If God wants to heal me, He will do it without using any medicine." And when the health of some of them deteriorated, they started to blame God, and sometimes they even questioned their faith. For me, that is not faith. If you are giving God just one way to work, you may be perceiving God as a miracle performer. What if that was not what He wanted for you? You can't give Him conditions and guidelines to do His work. You must be open to His ways and to His will for your life. Be open to what he wants you to learn during your journey.

Is that true? Doing things our own way could delay God's plans for us?

Moses wanted to serve the Lord in his own way when he was young and a healthy man. It was the perfect time for Moses, but God wanted him for a very specific big mission. He wanted him to be a wise and patient man. God didn't go searching for another person who had these specifications ready for this mission. Instead, He took all the time needed and the hard work to shape Moses to be the perfect man for the mission.

It took him 40 years to be that man. I think Moses himself had given up on believing that one day he could do anything that he had wanted 40 years before. He became old and his tongue was heavy. But, from God's perspective, Moses became the perfect man for the mission. After 40 years, God could finally start doing wonders with Moses. In this journey, Moses became humble and teachable to finally become the man that God could depend on.

On the other hand, because of their stubbornness and insisting on doing everything their own way, the people of Israel rejected God's way. The path that should have taken a few months took them 40 whole years to finish—to get to the promised land. Not just that, a whole generation didn't even have the chance to see it. Their actions made the Lord revoke His promise for them. They delayed God's plans, promises, and blessings.

God's plans depend on you, how humble you are and how far you are willing to let Him work to shape your character to be in harmony with His ways. Even in the time of pain. So, trust his plans, believe in yourself, and remember that *YOUR PAIN IS NOT A WASTE.*

The End

Acknowledgments

Remon, Pharmacist, Husband, Amazing Caregiver
I must start by thanking my amazing husband, Remon. What you did for me is beyond any words I could ever say. Without your love and support, I couldn't have gone this far. You taught me how love can endure. Your presence helped me fight. Your support enabled me to achieve my dream. To be who I am today is because of you and your unconditional love.

Judy Watters, Writing Consultant/Editor
Hearts Need Art
There are no words to describe how thankful and grateful I am for your huge help to me while writing this book. You cared about this book as if it were your own. Your encouragement gave me all the confidence and the support I needed to keep writing. Thanks for the hours you spent reading and editing. Thanks for providing advice and layout options for this book to be in the best shape.

Susan Wandishin, LifeList Coordinator
Dear Jack Foundation
I am very thankful to the Dear Jack Foundation. Who made my wish come true. And special thanks for Susan Wandishin who worked so hard to

connect me with the perfect people in every step.

Maxwell Mitzel, Final Editor
Thanks for helping in reviewing and editing. Thanks for your dedication and commitment to the deadlines and for handling the last few weeks' pressure to get it done on time.

Sandy Saleeb, Translator of Neveen's and Mays's Chapters
Thanks so much to Sandy, my best friend, for transcribing Neveen's and May's stories. Thanks for the precious time we spent in Zoom meetings working and laughing. Thanks for calming me down when I got stressed out.

Moffitt Cancer Center
So thankful for Dr. R and his team for their care and support. For not giving up on my case. For being the best in the field and for providing top notch medical care and treatment. You made me feel like I was your only patient. Thanks to Adolescent and Young Adult (AYA) with cancer program that cares for the patient's emotional side while the medical team cares for their health.

My Family and Friends
Mom, Dad, Neveen, Magued, Mirna, Mays, John,

and Deena. You have been with me the whole way. Thanks for every prayer and the love you provided. You were a great support for me even with the long distance between us.

My friend and my doctor, Viviane
Thanks for encouraging me to write this book while I still had cancer and receiving chemo. I remember your words that I must write what I feel even if it seemed like there was no hope because those memories are too precious to be lost.

Thanks to those who didn't know me personally but supported me through prayer as we fought this battle together. You made me feel that I have a very big family that I never met but always felt their love.

God's Perfect Timing
Judy Sheer Watters
Writing Consultant
YOUR PAIN IS NOT A WASTE

God truly does work His plan for our lives in tiny wondrous miracles every step of the way. He worked in my life to give me the blessings of meeting Dalia, Remon, and the opportunity to help bring their story to many hurting people.

1. The publisher of my first book passed away suddenly in July of 2015. John was a very sweet Christian man who I loved dearly. His wife asked me to take over ownership of her husband's publishing business.

2. After much prayer, I did acquire John's business in December of 2015 and immediately started working with many authors.

3. Through one of the authors, my name was given to the founder of Hearts Need Art (HNA), a non-profit organization who at that time, offered music and visual art to cancer patients and their loved ones at the Methodist Hospital in San Antonio.

4. HNA contacted me to develop a writing

program for them. I started working with HNA in June of 2019 and visiting with cancer patients and their loved ones every Monday helping them to write through their journey.

5. Because I worked with HNA, I was asked to teach a seminar for Adolescent and Young Adult (AYA) Oncology caregivers conference in February 2020.

6. Through that seminar, a caregiver with the Dear Jack Foundation asked me if she might contact me later in reference to helping a cancer patient to fulfill her wish of writing her story.

And some people say modern-day miracles don't happen. What if I had never moved to San Antonio? What if I had written one book and stopped? What if I had taken my book to a different publisher? What if I had never heard of HNA? What if…? What if…? The list goes on.

I believe that God prepared me for "such a time as this" and for *Dalia's* book. God *does* work in mysterious ways to fulfill His design for our lives and to show His love for us through these blessings. I have been blessed by Dalia's story and by Remon's never-ending love for her. And now you have been blessed likewise.